PROBLEMS OF BLOOD PRESSURE IN CHILDHOOD

Publication Number 463
AMERICAN LECTURE SERIES®

A Monograph in
AMERICAN LECTURES IN PEDIATRICS

Edited by

JOHN A. ANDERSON, M.D.

Professor and Head
Department of Pediatrics
University of Minnesota Medical School
Minneapolis, Minnesota

Problems of Blood Pressure in Childhood

By

ARTHUR J. MOSS, M.D.

Associate Professor of Pediatrics (Cardiology)
Department of Pediatrics
University of California School of Medicine
Los Angeles, California

and

FORREST H. ADAMS, M.D.

Professor of Pediatrics and Head
Division of Cardiology, Department of Pediatrics
University of California School of Medicine
Los Angeles, California

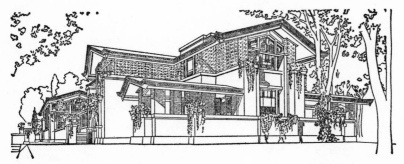

CHARLES C THOMAS • PUBLISHER

Springfield • *Illinois* • *U.S.A.*

CHARLES C THOMAS • PUBLISHER

BANNERSTONE HOUSE

301-327 East Lawrence Avenue, Springfield, Illinois, U.S.A.

*With THOMAS BOOKS careful attention is given to all details of
manufacturing and design. It is the Publisher's desire to present books
that are satisfactory as to their physical qualities and artistic possibilities
and appropriate for their particular use. THOMAS BOOKS will be true
to those laws of quality that assure a good name and good will.*

Printed in the United States of America

PREFACE

Estimation of arterial blood pressure in infants and children has now become a common office and hospital procedure. Coincident with this increasing interest, however, a dearth of information continues to exist relative to certain aspects of arterial pressure in children. This fact together with a conflict of some of the ideas expressed in the literature has served as the stimulus for the present effort.

The purpose in mind is to present some of the significant background information, as well as the existing data relevant to the methodology and interpretation of arterial pressure measurements in the pediatric age group. The monograph is by no means intended as a complete reference for the many extensive ramifications of the broad subject of arterial blood pressure in humans.

The contents embody a brief review of the history of arterial pressure measurements and a discussion of the current methods of estimation and the range of normal values. The final chapter deals with physiologic interpretation of the available data. Present evidence derived from animal and human observations does not yet permit complete comprehension of the features of arterial pressure which are peculiar to childhood. This represents a striking void in our knowledge, and the need for further research in this area is emphasized.

ACKNOWLEDGMENTS

This work was supported (in part) by Public Health Service research and training grants (H-5810, 2A-5292 and HTS-5449) from the Division of Research Grants, the National Institute of Arthritis and Metabolic Diseases, and the National Heart Institute, Public Health Service.

Grateful acknowledgement is made to Dr. John M. Adams, Professor and Chairman of the Department of Pediatrics, and to Dr. Victor Hall, Professor of Physiology, University of California School of Medicine, Los Angeles, for critically reading the manuscript. We are also grateful for assistance received from Dr. David Saxon, Professor of Physics, University of California, Los Angeles, and to Dr. Wilfrid Dixon, Professor of Preventive Medicine and Public Health (Biostatistics), Mrs. Muriel Huggins, Senior Statistician, Dr. Bernard J. O'Loughlin, Professor of Radiology, and Dr. Wilbert Liebling, Assistant Clinical Professor of Pediatrics, all of the University of California School of Medicine, Los Angeles.

A.J.M.

F.H.A.

CONTENTS

PROBLEMS OF BLOOD PRESSURE
IN CHILDHOOD

Chapter I

THE HISTORY OF
BLOOD PRESSURE MEASUREMENT

Mamometric methods of blood pressure measurement as we recognize them today did not appear suddenly upon the medical horizon but developed gradually from a series of contributions made throughout the years by numerous physicians and physiologists. Earliest amongst these was the Reverend Stephen Hales[1] who in 1733 successfully measured the arterial pressure of the blood within the artery of a horse.

In Hales[1] earliest experiments he inserted a glass tube vertically into the artery of a horse and measured the distance that the blood rose within the tube. These experiments are probably best described in his own words: "In December, I caused a mare to be tied down alive on her back; she was 14 hands high, and about 14 years of age, had a fistula on her withers, was neither very lean nor yet lusty: having laid open the left crural artery about 3 inches from her belly, I inserted into it a brass pipe whose bore was one-sixth of an inch in diameter; and to that, by means of another brass pipe which was fitly adapted to it, I fixed a glass tube, of nearly the same diameter, which was 9 feet in length: then untying the ligature on the artery, the blood rose in the tube 8 feet 3 inches perpendicular above the level of the left ventricle of the heart, but it did not attain to its full height at once: it rushed up about half-way in an instant, and afterwards gradually at each pulse 12, 8, 6, 4, 2 and sometimes 1 inch: when it was at its full height, it would rise and fall at and after each pulse 2, 3 or 4 inches; sometimes it would fall 12 to 14 inches and have there for a time the same vibrations up and down, at and after each pulse, as it had, when it was at its full height; to which it would rise again, after forty or fifty pulses."

Hales estimated the pressure of the blood in man to be about

7½ feet which is a remarkably close approximation when one considers the crudeness of his technique.

The piezometer tube of Hales was replaced almost a century later (1828) when Poiseuille[2,3] introduced the mercury manometer. This apparatus consisted of a U tube filled at one end with mercury and at the other with an anticoagulent solution of subcarbonate of soda. The arm containing the anticoagulant solution was inserted directly into the artery of an animal, and the intra-arterial pressure was then transmitted to the mercury column. Because of the excessive weight of the mercury, however, the reading obtained with this instrument more closely approximated the mean than the systolic and diastolic extremes of pressure.

The first recorded blood pressure measurement was made by Ludwig[4] in the year 1847. Utilizing a kymograph, he was able to record on a revolving drum the movements of the mercury column of a Poiseuille manometer.

None of these early attempts at intra-arterial blood pressure measurement could be applied to man, but there subsequently followed a period of gradual evolution which ultimately did lead to the development of manometer systems capable of registering in man the two extremes of a pulsating pressure.[5-16]

The first indirect estimation of blood pressure was accomplished by Karl Vierordt[17] in 1855 who devised a sphygmomanometer which recorded the radial artery pulsations on a kymograph. By the ingenious use of a complex weight system, this instrument crudely measured the level of the systolic blood pressure. The measurement was based upon the amount of weight which was necessary to obliterate the radial pulsations.

In the years to follow, Marey[18-20] and others[21-23] constructed similar manometers based upon this same principle. However, these also were extremely crude instruments, and the results obtained with their use were grossly inaccurate.

It was not until 1875 that, owing largely to Marey's efforts, a reasonably accurate apparatus was introduced. It was also during this period that Marey,[24] Mosso,[25] and Gaertner[26] independently developed manometers for the estimation of the digital blood pressure.

Gaertner's digital manometer consisted of a pneumatic cuff which could be applied to the finger and inflated, thereby rendering the finger bloodless. With gradual deflation of the cuff, the blood returned and a distinct flush occurred. The appearance of the flush was regarded as the end-point and was interpreted as representing the systolic pressure of the arterial blood. This technique was actually the forerunner of the flush method for the measurement of blood pressure in infants as introduced in 1952.[27,28]

Estimation of blood pressure by palpation is the oldest of the clinically acceptable methods of indirect measurement. Based upon the preliminary findings of others,[21,29,30] it was introduced by Riva-Rocci in 1896.[33,34] The method, as he employed it, consisted of compression of the arm with a pneumatic cuff which was inflated by a rubber bulb. The pressure in the cuff was registered on a mercury or aneroid manometer, and with gradual decompression the radial pulsations became palpable. The level at which these pulsations first appeared was assumed to represent the systolic blood pressure.

The oscillatory or visual method of measuring blood pressure as it is practiced today was first introduced by Erlanger[35] in the year 1904. This method is based upon the visualization of oscillations transmitted by the arterial pulsations to the mercury column of the manometer. Many modifications of the original procedure have since been introduced, and a number of oscillometers are now available commercially.[36,37] For the most part, however, their use is restricted to investigational studies or to observations in adults suffering from peripheral vascular disease.

The evolution of auscultatory manometry constitutes one of the most interesting chapters in the development of blood pressure techniques. It had its inception in the year 1905 when Korokoff, a Russian physician, first advocated this method of measurement. Korotkoff's observations were reported at a meeting of the Imperial Military Medical Academy in St. Petersburg, in December of that year.[38-41] A full translation reads as follows:

"On the basis of his observation, the speaker came to the conclusion that a perfectly constructed artery under normal conditions does not emit any sounds. Taking this fact into consideration, the speaker proposes the sound method for measuring blood pressure on human beings. The sleeve of Riva-Rocci is put on the middle third of the arm; the pressure in this sleeve rises rapidly until the circulation below this sleeve stops completely. At first there are no sounds whatsoever. As the mercury in the manometer drops to a certain height, there appear the first short or faint tones, the appearance of which indicates that part of the pulse wave of the blood stream has passed under the sleeve. Consequently, the reading on the manometer when the first sound appears corresponds to the maximum blood pressure; with the further fall of the mercury in the manometer, there are heard systolic pressure murmurs which again become sounds (secondary). Finally all sounds disappear. The time of the disappearance of the sounds indicates the free passage or flow of the blood stream; in other words, at the moment of the disappearance or fading out of the sounds, the minimum blood pressure in the artery has surpassed the pressure in the sleeve. Consequently, the reading of the manometer at this time corresponds to the minimum blood pressure. Experiments conducted on animals gave positive results. The first sound tones appear (10-12 mm.) sooner than the pulse which (1. ar. radialis) can be felt only after the passage of the major portion of the blood stream."

The technique described by Korotkoff was rapidly accepted and soon came into widespread use. Despite numerous critical re-evaluations, his original concept is still tenable — a testimony to the sound caliber of his thinking.

Since Korotkoff's original contribution, there has actually been little progress in the field of clinical sphygmomanometry. Those advances which have occurred have been limited almost entirely to the intra-arterial method of measurement.

SUMMARY

Blood pressure measurement was first accomplished more than two centuries ago by the intra-arterial method. Since its inauguration, blood pressure manometry has undergone a gradual evolution. As practiced today, it is the product of a prolonged series of observations made by numerous physicians and physiologists.

REFERENCES

1. Hales, S.: *Statical Essays*: Containing Haemastaticks; or an account of some hydraulick and hydrostatical experiments made on the blood and blood vessels of animals, London, Innys and Manby, 1733.

2. Poiseuille, J. L. M.: Recherches sur la force du coeur aortique, *J. de physiol. exper., Par., 8*:272, 1828.

3. Poiseuille, J. L. M.: Recherches sur la force du coeur aortique, *J. de physiol. exper., Par., 9*:341, 1829.

4. Ludwig, C. F. W.: Beiträge zur Kenntnis des Einflusses der Respirations-bewegungen auf Blutlauf im Aortensystem, *Arch. Anat. Physiol. wiss. Med.,* 242, 1847.

5. Hürthle, K.: Beiträge zur hämadynamik. Erste abhaudlung: zur technik der Untersuchung des Blutdrickes, *Arch. F. d. ges. Physiol., 43*:399, 1888.

6. Frank, O.: Ein neues optisches Federmanometer, *Ztschr. f. Biol., 82*:49, 1925.

7. Wiggers, C. J., and Baker, W. R.: A new universal optical manometer, *J. Lab. and Clin. Med., 10*:54, 1924.

8. Hamilton, W. F., Brewer, J., and Brotman, I.: Pressure pulse contours in the intact animal. Analytical description of a new high-frequency hypodermic manometer with illustrative curves of simultaneous arterial and intracardiac pressures, *Am. J. Physiol., 107*:427, 1934.

9. Gregg, D. E., Eckstein, R. W., and Feinberg, M. H.: Pressure pulses and blood pressure values in unanesthetized dogs, *Am. J. Physiol., 118*, 399, 1937.

10. Beyne, J., and Gougerot, L.: Une méthode de transmission électrique et d'enregistrement á distance de la pression arteriélle et du débit respiratoire, *Compt. rend. Soc. de biol., 131*:770, 1939.

11. Golberg, H., and Eyster, J. A. E.: Relation of contraction of different regions of ventricle of the turtle to rise of intraventricular pressure, *Am. J. Physiol., 131*:416, 1940.

12. Gomez, D. M.: *Hemodynamique et Angiocinetique;* Etude rationelle des lois regissant les phenomenes cardiovasculaires, Paris, Hermann, 1941.

13. Hampel, A.: Elektrisches transmissionsmanometer auf der grundlage *Arch. f. d. ges. Physiol., 244*:171, 1940. elektrischer widerstandsanderungen des wismuts im magnetfeld

14. Rein, H.: Photoelektrisches transmissions - manometer zur blutdruck-schreibung, *Arch. f. d. ges. Physiol., 243*:329, 1940.

15. Green, H. D.: Circulation: Physical Principles,   In Glasser, O. (Ed.) : *Medical Physics,* Chicago, Year Book Publishers, 1944.

16. Green, H. D.: Circulatory System: Methods, In Glasser, O. (Ed.) : *Medical Physics,* Chicago, Year Book Publishers, 1950.

17. Vierordt, K.: Die lehre vom arterienpuls in gesunden und kraulsen zustäuden. Gegrundet auf eine neue methode der bildlichen darstellung des menschlichen pulses, Braunschweig, F. Vieweg U. Sohn, 1855.

18. Marey, E. J.: Recherches sur le pouls au moyen d'un nouvel appareil enregistreur, le sphygmograph, *Gaz. med. de Par. 3 s., 15*:225, 236, 298, 1860.

19. Marey, E. J.: *La Methode Graphique dans les Sciences Experimentales et Principalement en Physiologie et en Medicine,* Paris, Masson, 1878.

20. Marey, E. J.: *La Circulation du Sang a l'état Physiologique et dans les Maladies,* Paris, Masson, 1881.

21. Foster, B. W.: Note on the regulation of the pressure on the artery in the application of the sphygmograph, Brit. and For. M. - Chir. Rev., *40*:240, 1867.

22. Landlois, L.: Die Lehre vom Arterienpuls nach eigenenVersuchen und Beobachtungen dargestellt, Berlin, Hirschwald, 1872.

23. Philadelphian, A.: Le sphygmometrograph, *Compt. rend. Soc de biol. 10s., 3*:199, 1896.

24. Marey, E. J.: Nouvelles Recherches sur la Mesure Manometrique de la Pression du Sang chez L'homme, In his Physiol. exp., Paris, Masson, 1880.

25. Mosso, A.: Sphygmomanometre pour mesurer la pression du sang chez l'homme, *Arch. Ital. de biol., 23*:177, 1895.

26. Gaertner, G.: Ueber einen neuen Blutdruckmesser (tonomoter), *Wien Klin. Wchnschr., 12*:696, 1899.

27. Cappe, B. E., and Pallin, I. M.: Systolic blood pressure determination in the newborn and infant, *Anesthesiology, 13*:648, 1952.

28. Goldring, D., and Wohltmann, H.: Flush method for blood pressure determinations in newborn infants, *J. Pediat., 40*:285, 1952.

29. Behier: Un nouveau sphygmograph perfectionne de M. Longuet, *Bull. Acad. de med., Par., 33*:962, 1868.

30. Landois, L.: *Traité de Physiologie Humaine,* Trad. sur la 7 éd. Allemande par G. Moquin-Tandon, Paris, Reinwald, 1893.

31. von Basch, S.: UUeber die Messung des Blutdruckes am Menschen, *Ztshr. f. klin. Med., 2*:79, 1880.

32. Potain, P. C. E.: La pression artérielle de l'homme á létat normal et pathologique, Paris, Masson, 1902.

33. Riva-Rocci, S.: Un nuovo sfigmomanometro, *Gass. med di torino, 47*:981, 1896.

34. Riva-Rocci, S.: Per la misura della pressione arteriosa nell' nomo, *Gass. med. di torino, 1*:481, 1899.

35. Erlanger, J.: A new instrument for determining the minimum and maximum blood pressures in man, *Johns Hopkins Hosp. Rep., 12*:53, 1904.

36. Christensen, B. C.: Oscillometric studies; change of sensitivity of the oscillometer at the different pressures, and on the influence of the state of contraction of the arterial wall on the oscillometric curve, *Acta Med. Scandin., 120*:474, 1945.

37. Ejrup, B.: Tonoscillography after exercise; A new method for early diagnosis of organic arterial disease leading to intermittent claudication and for differential diagnosis of organic and functional arterial diseases with a special type of apparatus adapted to this purpose, *Acta med. Scandinav., 130*:1-suppl. 211, 1948.

38. Korotkoff, N. S.: On methods of studying blood pressure, Izviest. Imp. Voyenno-Med. *Akad. S.-Peterb., 11*:365, 1905.

39. Pickering, G. W.: *High Blood Pressure*, London, Churchill, 1955.

40. Lewis, W. H., Jr.: The evolution of clinical sphygmomanometry, *Bull. New York Acad. Med., 17*:871, 1941.

41. Gittings, J. C.: Auscultatory blood pressure determinations; a preliminary report, *Arch. Int. Med., 6*:196, 1910.

Chapter II

THE INDIRECT METHODS OF
BLOOD PRESSURE MEASUREMENT

Arterial pressure may be measured indirectly by a variety of methods. Regardless of the method used, it is quite important that the examiner be aware of the many factors which may affect the reading obtained. Reported observations, for example, suggest that there may be a significant difference in blood pressure between individuals, depending among other things upon racial origin, climatic environment and daily dietary habits.[1-8] Of greater importance to the clinician, perhaps, is the recognition that at all ages there may be considerable variation in blood pressure in the same individual — even from heart beat to heart beat.

During the course of 24 hours the arterial blood pressure undergoes considerable variation. The systolic pressure has been observed to vary diurnally with a low point in the early morning hours and a high point in the early evening hours.[9-10] At complete rest, as with sound sleep, the systolic pressure is reduced. After meals, slight transient increases in blood pressure have been noted.[9]

A rise in blood pressure may occur as a result of strong sensory stimuli or of reflexes originating in a distended urinary bladder. Exercise, because of its effect upon cardiac output, will cause a transient rise in the systolic blood pressure.[11]

Tilting a subject from the supine to the erect position has been shown to have little effect upon blood pressure.[12,13] It is likely that the hydrostatic effects resulting from changes in position are counteracted by vascular reflexes.

A number of other factors are known to affect the arterial pressure. Physiologic factors,[14] such as fear and apprehension or exposure to cold, tend to raise the arterial pressure. Exposure to heat, on the other hand, tends to reduce the pressure.

Physiologic periodic undulations in blood pressure which

may be as great as 40 mm. Hg are believed to occur and have been referred to as Traube waves, Hering waves, Traube-Hering waves, Mayer waves, vasomotor waves, interference waves or third order waves.[15] It is not yet known whether these waves are due to periodic variation in vasomotor activity, to changes in the heart rate and stroke volume or to the respiratory movements.

It should be recognized that the procedure of blood pressure measurement in itself involves certain physiological alterations which may exert an effect upon the arterial pressure; i.e., compression of the vessels, cutaneous stimulation and the changing emotions of the subject.

It is apparent then that the level of arterial blood pressure is influenced by a large number of factors, some of which may be extremely difficult or even impossible to control. Because of the extreme variability and complexity of these factors, the optimal conditions for blood pressure measurement are difficult to delineate. The closest approach, probably, is under basal conditions when physical and mental rest is complete. Although feasible for investigational studies, such conditions can hardly be considered practical for routine clinical use.

GENERAL PRECAUTIONS

The Patient

Even in the basal state, both the systolic and diastolic pressures may vary significantly with the phase of respiration or the phase of blood flow. These differences are greatly magnified by deep breathing or by changes in the rate or rhythm of the heart. Thus crying, laughing, giggling, apprehension, emotional stress, previous activity and abnormal body temperatures may profoundly affect the level of blood pressure.

Whenever possible, efforts should be made to approach basal conditions by reassuring the child and allowing time for recovery from apprehension or recent activity. The state of relaxation of an infant or child who is awake may change from moment to moment and no doubt accounts for a part of the extreme variation sometimes obtained with consecutive readings.

The Instrument

A frequent source of error is the instrument itself. In selecting the manometer, a careful inspection for mechanical defects should be made. The component parts are examined for leaks, and it should be established that the valve functions smoothly and efficiently. In the case of a mercury manometer, dirty tubes and oxidation of mercury may produce a poor meniscus; loss of mercury may displace the zero level.

The aneroid manometer is probably inferior to the mercury type apparatus since mechanical hysteresis tends to cause a loss in linearity which may result in gross inaccuracies. When this instrument is used it is essential to stimultaneously compare pressures at various levels with those registered by a mechanically perfect mercury manometer. This can be accomplished by at-

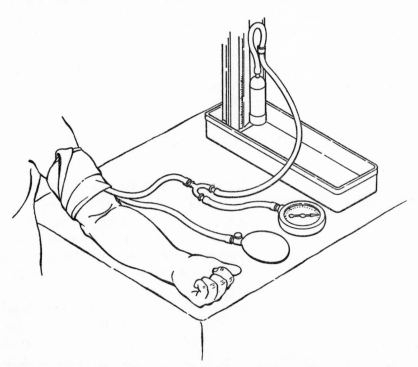

Fig. 1. Diagram illustrating a method for establishing the accuracy of an aneroid manometer. Pressure registrations are compared simultaneously with those of a mechanically perfect mercury manometer by attaching the two manometers to a single arm cuff.

taching one tube of the compression bag to a Y connector which in turn is attached to the two manometers (Fig. 1).

Technique of Measurement

Errors in measurement are frequently the result of improper technique. For precise readings certain precautions are essential. The mercury column must be vertical, and the observer's eye should be level with the meniscus. It is important to select a cuff of appropriate width since one too large or too small may give rise to a significant error. The cuff must be applied to the bare arm evenly and snugly and should be inflated rapidly and deflated slowly at a rate of about 5 mm. Hg per second. Before additional determinations are made, the cuff should be completely deflated.

The Operator

For the most accurate results, it is recommended that the average of at least two determinations of systolic and diastolic pressure be recorded as the final reading. If the physician suffers auditory impairment, he might profit from the use of an electronic stethescope since the sounds in children may be exceedingly faint. Measurement of blood pressure should not be entrusted to personnel with insufficient auscultatory experience since auditory acuity improves with training.

BLOOD PRESSURE MEASUREMENT BY AUSCULTATION

Knowledge of the pressure of the blood within the arterial system may be gained by a variety of clinical and laboratory procedures. For clinical purposes, the most commonly used method today is that of auscultation. This consists of the auscultatory detection and interpretation of vascular sounds induced in an artery by proximal constriction with an air-pressure arm cuff. The method is generally applicable to all age groups with the exception of early infancy where the vascular sounds are usually so feeble and indistinct that accurate interpretation is not possible.

Technique

Whenever possible, sufficient time should be allowed for recovery from apprehension, meals or exercise. The child may be placed in either a recumbent or sitting position. The arm should be perfectly relaxed in a position of slight flexion and abduction. If the measurement is made with the patient in a sitting position, the forearm should be supported on a smooth surface at the level of the heart. The sphygmomanometer cuff should be applied evenly and snugly about the bared arm. The lower edge of the cuff should be about one inch above the antecubital space (Fig. 2).

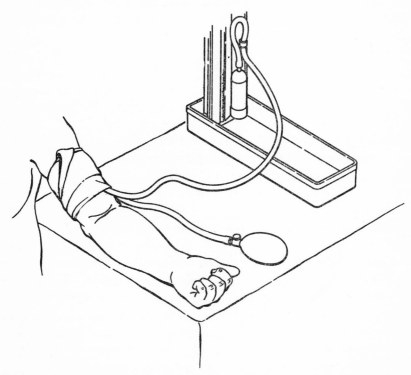

Fig. 2. Diagram showing arm position and sphygmomanometer cuff application. The cuff should be applied evenly and snugly about the bared arm, the lower edge being about one inch above the antecubital space. The forearm should be in a position of slight flexion and abduction and must be at the level of the heart.

The manometer need not be placed at heart level. It is important, however, to check the accuracy of the instrument, to place the mercury column in a vertical position and to read the meniscus at eye level. It is often helpful to first locate the course of the artery in the antecubital space by palpation. The stethescope receiver can then be applied firmly to this area but must be free from contact with the lower edge of the cuff. Slight variation in pressure may be necessary to improve the quality and distinctness of the sounds.

The cuff should be inflated rapidly, but it is recommended that the system be deflated slowly at a rate of about 5 mm. Hg. per second. If the release of pressure is too rapid, the reading will be inaccurate on the low side. The rate of inflation of the cuff is also of importance. If it is too slow, the arm veins become congested, and the level at which the first sounds appear is lowered. In addition, there is apt to occur a short period between systole and diastole during which all sounds completely disappear (auscultatory gap).[16,17] If the auscultatory gap does occur or if there are signs of venous congestion, the procedure should be repeated. If the arm veins are congested before inflation, then the cuff should be inflated while the arm is upraised.

When the cuff of the sphygmomanometer is applied to the upper arm and inflated, the soft tissues directly beneath the cuff are compressed. If the pressure within the cuff exceeds the peak pressure of the arterial pulse wave, the artery is completely occluded, and the pulse wave cannot penetrate. With gradual release of pressure, a point is reached at which the vessel begins to open, and the peak of the pulse wave is transmitted to the periphery. At this level distinctive vascular sounds (Korotkoff sounds) become audible through a stethescope applied in the antecubital space over the distal part of the artery.

There are four phases of sound which make their appearance as the pressure in the arm cuff is gradually reduced:

Phase I   — Distinct but ususally faint sounds suddenly appear.

Phase II — The sounds of Phase I become prolonged into a murmur.

Phase III— The sounds increase in intensity.

Phase IV — The sounds decrease in intensity and
    finally disappear.

Some prefer to separate the final disappearance of sounds
and classify them as a fifth phase.

The lack of accord amongst various authorities regarding
interpretation of the induced arterial sounds has been a source
of confusion. Korotkoff initially recommended that the beginning
of the first sound phase be taken as the index of the systolic pressure and the end of the fourth phase (complete disappearance of
sounds) as the index of the diastolic pressure. Although there
has been general agreement on the first point, the phase for determining the diastolic level has remained controversial.

In 1939, a joint committee of the American Heart Association
and the Cardiac Society of Great Britain and Ireland agreed that
the diastolic pressure should be read at a point where the sounds
abruptly begin to fade (onset of phase IV). They further recommended that if the sounds disappear at a lower level, this also
should be recorded.

In July, 1951, a committee functioning under the auspices
of the American Heart Association[18,19] concluded that the point
of complete disappearance of sounds is the best index of the
diastolic pressure, and the point of muffling should be accepted
only in those cases where the auscultatory sounds persist to zero.
Their revision was made on the following grounds:

"(A) The current practice of using the point of sudden
muffling of the sounds was based (1) on comparisons with oscillatory criteria, and (2) on hemodynamic data derived from
studies of excised or isolated arteries undergoing direct compression or decompression. The former (1) is of dubious value since
no general agreement has been reached regarding the oscillatory
criteria of diastolic pressure. The latter (2) appears to be risky
owing to the fact that unsolved physical factors may enter when
pressure is transferred to arteries from a cuff of arbitrary size
through the tissues of a limb.

"(B) While some difficulties still exist in making absolute
comparisons between pressures determined by optical manometers and those revealed by auscultatory criteria, a limited number of such comparisons strongly suggests that, on the average,

the cessation of sounds conforms rather better to the intra-arterial diastolic pressure and that dulling of sounds appears 5 to 10 mm. Hg. above this level.

"(C) Accuracy, not applicability to every individual, should determine the choice of criteria. The fact that sounds may persist as cuff pressure is reduced to lower levels, or even to zero, in certain clinical states, such as aortic insufficiency, hyperthyroidism, anemia, and in an occasional normal person, should not determine the selection of an equivalent criterion for diastolic pressure if it is not exact. The fact remains that cessation of sounds does occur in a very large percentage of all individuals examined. It is therefore recommended that the less exact criterion of muffled sounds be used only when necessary and that such readings be recorded as the point of muffled sounds. If any significance is attached to the fact that sounds are heard below this point, it should be recorded.

"(D) Tests of different examiners reveal that, probably owing to different degrees of auditory acuity, there is a greater uniformity in decisions as to when sounds cease than as to the point at which they begin to muffle. Hence, greater uniformity in recording diastolic pressures and enhancement of their accuracy in any statistical study may be expected by using disappearance of sounds as a criterion. Furthermore, the distinctness or demarcation of the dulling phase varies in different subjects examined. Frankness must cause us to admit that all too frequently the reading of diastolic pressure by this criterion becomes merely a guess."

In a stimulating review, Burton[20] considered these recommendations "a major setback to medical science" and presented cogent evidence favoring the muffling of sounds over their disappearance as the criterion for the diastolic level. The issue remains unsettled as of this writing. Comparative studies using direct measurements as a "baseline" have, in our hands, been most disappointing. By either method, correlation was so poor that there was little from which to choose. Our experience indicates that at best auscultatory estimation of diastolic pressure is a grossly inaccurate measurement.

Origin of the Korotkoff Sounds

The mechanism whereby the induced vascular sounds arise is not yet known. Throughout the years several explanations have been advanced. These may be listed as follows: (1) sudden expansion of the vessel wall,[21,22] (2) the "water hammer" phenomenon,[23,24,25] (3) the "pre-anacrotic phenomenon"[26,27] (4) the "Bernoulli effect,"[22,28] and (5) turbulence of blood flow.[29,30]

(1) Sudden expansion of the vessel wall as the cause of the induced vascular sounds was first proposed by Korotkoff.[21] This hypothesis embodies the concept that as the pressure in the arm cuff is gradually reduced, the primary pulsation forces apart the relaxed wall of the collapsed artery distal to the cuff. The sound is believed to result from the sudden sharp stretching of the arterial wall.

(2) The "water hammer" hypothesis was proposed by Erlanger[24] in 1916. The term "water hammer" refers to the pressure which is exerted when the motion of a volume of fluid suddenly meets resistance. These pressure effects may indeed be extremely powerful. The concept maintains that with release of vascular compression a large volume of blood flows with considerable velocity into the opening artery. When this meets the sluggish or stationary column of blood in the distal uncompressed portion, the "water hammer" effect is produced. The resultant pressure causes the arterial wall to vibrate, and the vibration produces the sound.

(3) In 1920, Erlanger presented evidence which suggested that a prominent factor in the production of the Korotkoff sounds is what he termed the "pre-anacrotic phenomenon." This view contends that as the constricted vessel is decompressed, a negative wave immediately precedes the anacrotic limb of the arterial pulse. It is present from the time the pulse first penetrates to the beginning of the fourth sound phase. It was postulated that these pre-anacrotic waves, by exerting a sudden shock on the wall of the vessel, are the source of the vascular sounds.

(4) The "Bernoulli effect" is a term used to denote a decrease in lateral pressure as the velocity of a volume of fluid increases. Since the artery directly under the pressure cuff is partially constricted, the blood as it flows through the stenotic portion must

increase in velocity. This results in a reduction of lateral pressure at the constricted site, and the walls of the vessel tend to become more collapsed. As the process continues, the vessel becomes almost completely occluded, and the velocity approaches zero. All of the energy of the column then becomes available as lateral pressure, and the walls of the vessel are blown apart. As the process repeats itself, an intermittent type of flow develops with resultant wall vibration.

(5) Lange and his associates[29] suggested in 1956 that turbulence of flow is responsible for the production of the Korotkoff sounds. They hypothesized that the rapid changes in the vascular diameter are associated with changes in velocity profile and that a turbulent flow pattern is thereby produced. Turbulent flow is characterized by secondary irregular motions with crossing of flow lines and eddies. By liberation of energy, this can be a source of sound. When the energy is completely dissipated, a laminar flow pattern is re-established. The situation is analagous to the "hydraulic-jump" in which two laminar flow patterns at different mean velocities and cross-sectional areas are separated by turbulent flow and energy loss.

It is possible that two or more of the aforementioned factors may operate together. Thus, Rappaport and Luisada[22] suggest that factors (1) and (4) are responsible, whereas Malcolm[31] believes that factors (2) and (5) are involved.

Selection of the Cuff

Proper selection and application of the sphygmomanometer cuff is necessary for accurate results.[32-38] The pressure in the cuff is transmitted most effectively at its center, and if the cuff is of sufficient width, the pressure as indicated by the manometer penetrates to the artery itself. However, if the cuff is too narrow, the pressure within the cuff is poorly transmitted to the underlying artery, and the pressure recorded by the manometer is higher than that which exists within the artery (Fig. 3).

A cuff which is too wide is probably less productive of error than a cuff which is too narrow; however, some error may be assumed to occur even under these conditions. The longer segment of the compressed artery does cause a greater decrement

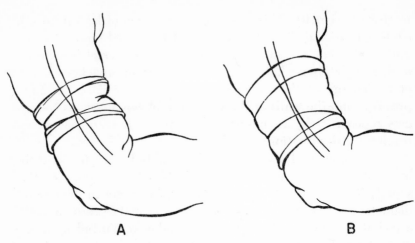

A   B

Fig. 3. Diagram showing the effect of an arm cuff which is too narrow. This results in poor transmission of the pressure to the underlying artery (A). The manometer reading in such a case is higher than the pressure which actually exists within the vessel. When a cuff of proper width is used, the pressure is effectively transmitted to the underlying artery (B) and more accurate readings are obtained.

in the pulse because of increased friction, and there is a tendency for the pulse to disappear before it reaches the lower edge of the cuff. This is reflected in a recorded arterial pressure which is lower than the true one. Nevertheless, the contention of Joos and his associates[39] that for practical purposes the largest size cuff is the least productive of error is probably correct.

Erroneous readings may also be obtained if the cuff is loosely applied.[40,41] This causes a ballooning of the bag with a narrowing of the effective cuff surface in contact with the tissues (Fig. 4). The result is a recorded arterial pressure which is greater than that which exists within the vessel.

Because of the major importance of the problem of cuff selection, the following study was conducted. Observations were made under basal conditions on 58 subjects ranging in age from one to 17 years. The majority had some type of congenital cardiac defect, but all were normotensive. Auscultatory measurements using cuffs of different widths (2.5 cm., 5 cm., 7 cm., 9.5 cm., and 12 cm.) were obtained in each subject except in occasional cases

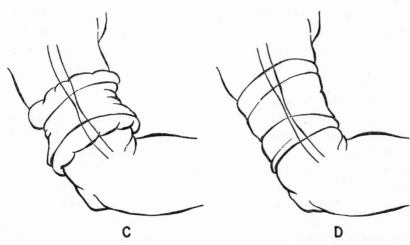

Fig. 4. Diagram showing the effect of a loosely applied arm cuff. With inflation, a ballooning of the cuff occurs, and the effective surface is narrowed (C). The manometer reading in this case is higher than that which actually exists within the vessel. When the cuff is snugly applied, ballooning does not occur, and the effective surface is not altered (D).

where the widest cuff was too large or the narrowest cuff too small for proper application. The systolic pressure was recorded as the very beginning of the first sound phase. In order to evaluate the diastolic index, both the point of muffling and the point of complete disappearance were recorded.

Immediately following the indirect determinations, direct pressure measurements were made in the brachial artery of the same arm. Under local infiltration with a 1 per cent solution of Xylocaine, the artery was exposed at the point of its bifurcation into the ulnar and radial branches. The vessels were perfused liberally with the 1 per cent Xylocaine solution to inhibit vascular spasm. A No. 19 arterial needle was introduced into the ulnar artery in such a manner that when fully advanced, its tip projected into the brachial artery. Using this method of cannulation, obstruction of the brachial artery by the needle itself was probably avoided.

The pressures were measured by a P23D Statham strain gauge and recorded by an Offner direct writing recorder. The natural frequency of the system when filled with distilled water at 24°C. was 100 cycles per second. This is more than adequate since Wood[42] has satisfactorily demonstrated that there is no significant difference in pressure levels recorded by different manometers systems with uniform response out to 6 cycles per second and above.

Since the 2.5 cm. cuff measurements could be obtained in only 28 of the subjects studied, data for this cuff were not included in the statistical analysis. Parameters recorded for each subject were age, weight, height, arm circumference and arm length. In addition, two ratios had been computed — weight/height and arm circumference/arm length. These seven variates are designated here as x_1, x_2 — x_7. For both systolic and diastolic readings, the differences between the measurements obtained by the direct method and by each of the measurements using the four cuff sizes were computed and designated as the dependent variates (Yj).

For the measurements of each cuff size, both systolic and diastolic, a linear regression equation of the form $Yj = B_0 + B_1x_1 + B_2x_2 + B_3x_3 + B_4x_4 + B_5x_5 + B_6x_6 + B_7x_7$ where the B i are the regression coefficients and Yj and the x_i are as previously stated. This equation enables one to predict what the estimated differences from the reading of the direct method would be for certain x_i values; that is, for a subject of a certain age, weight, height, etc.

Correlation coefficients were computed, giving measures of the relationships of the independent variates (x_i) with each other. Multiple correlation coefficients also were determined. Regression equations were obtained using the seven independent variates. Two of the independent variates were then selected, and a similar regression analysis was performed (for the systolic blood pressure measurements only) to yield regression equations which contained only the two independent variates. The object of this was to obtain a more practical means for adjusting blood pressure measurements than use of all seven variates. These regression problems were accomplished with the aid of the IBM 709 digital computer.

The correlation coefficients, giving measures of the relationships of the independent variates, x_i, with each other are presented in Table I. The interpretation of a high positive correlation coefficient is that the high values of one variable tend to be associated with the high values of the other, and the low values of one variable tend to be associated with the low values of the other.

TABLE I

CORRELATION COEFFICIENTS

		Age X_1	Weight X_2	Height X_3	Weight/ Height X_4	Arm Circum- ference X_5	Arm Length X_6	Arm Circum- ference/ Arm Length X_7
Age	X_1	1	.871	.942	.815	.623	.858	.470
Weight	X_2		1	.934	.984	.760	.861	.307
Height	X_3			1	.877	.661	.906	.501
Weight/Height	X_4				1	.784	.814	.210
Arm Circum- ference	X_5					1	.786	.114
Arm Length	X_6						1	.502
Arm Circumference/ Arm Length	X_7							1

The multiple correlation coefficient, R, gives a measure of the success of estimating the blood pressure adjustment using the estimating, or predicting, equation. The greater the agreement between the actual and the predicted values of the adjustment, Y, the higher will be the value of the multiple correlation coefficient, and thus the prediction power of the equation. The multiple correlation coefficients are presented in Table I. From these values it can be seen that the prediction power of the regression equations using the seven independent variates is greater for systolic than for diastolic measurements. In fact, it is so poor for diastolic measurements (regardless of the method used) that further statistical analysis was limited to the systolic measurements only.

Since the regression equations based on so many variates would be impractical for general usage in the adjustment of blood pressure measurements, it appeared to be desirable to reduce the number of variates in the equation. After inspection of the regression coefficients, the sums of squares of estimate and the multiple correlation coefficients, two variates were chosen to achieve the optimum reduction in the errors of estimate for two variates for systolic blood pressure measurements. The two variates chosen were height and arm circumference.

Regression analyses were performed on the data for the systolic measurements on the 58 subjects, and a new regression equation of the form $Yj = b_0 + b_3 x_3 + b_5 x_5$ was obtained for each cuff size.*

* $Yj =$ Blood pressure adjustment when cuff size j is used.
  $x_3 =$ Patient's height in cm.
  $x_5 =$ Patient's arm circumference in cm.

The multiple corelation coefficients obtained when only two variates were used are given in Table II.

It can be seen from this table that the value of R for the two-variate estimating equation is only slightly less than the value of R for the regression equation using all seven variates.

TABLE II

MULTIPLE CORRELATION COEFFICIENTS

	Cuff Size (Cm.)	R (7 variates)	R (2 variates)
Diastolic	5	.593	
	7	.397	
	9.5	.310	
	13	.237	
Systolic	5	.742	.685
	7	.658	.558
	9.5	.617	.541
	13	.566	.536

By substituting the various possible values for height and arm circumference in these regression equations, adjustment values were obtained and plotted. These adjustments represent numerical values to be either added to or subtracted from (depending upon the sign) the blood pressure reading obtained by using a particular cuff size. The adjusted blood pressure reading thus obtained is the best estimate of what the direct method would yield as a blood pressure measurement for an individual of a given height and arm circumference. A graph of these adjustment values for given heights and circumferences was prepared and is presented in Figure 5. The graph permits appropriate blood pressure adjustment for the particular cuff size which is used.

Figure 6 enables one to choose the cuff size requiring the

612.1 M855

SYSTOLIC BLOOD PRESSURE ADJUSTMENT ZONES FOR FOUR CUFF SIZES

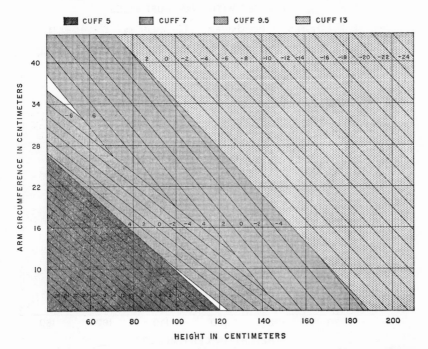

Fig. 5. Nomograph for adjusting the blood pressure reading when measured by auscultation. The adjustments are numerical values which depend upon the arm circumference and height of the individual and upon the size of the cuff used. The adjusted reading is an estimate of the intra-arterial systolic pressure.

least adjustment for a given height and arm circumference. For each cuff size, zones were determined which indicated the amount of adjustment to be made if the point of intersection of a patient's height and arm circumference falls therein. For example, for a height of 100 cm. and an arm circumference of 18 cm., cuff size seven would be chosen, and the blood pressure reading thus obtained would be adjusted by subtracting four from it. If, in this case, the blood pressure reading obtained were 118, adjustment of this reading would yield a value of 114.

The authors are well aware of the possible pitfalls of a study such as this. Because of physiologic "reactive errors," a comparison of the intra-arterial pressure to that recorded by auscultation

SYSTOLIC BLOOD PRESSURE ADJUSTMENT VALUES
FOR USE WITH FOUR CUFF SIZES

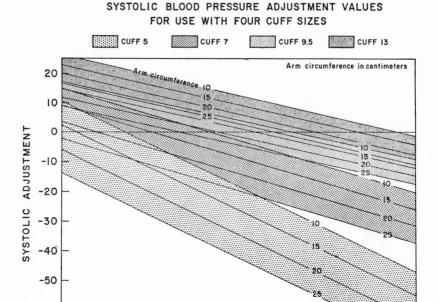

Fig. 6. Nomograph for selection of the appropriate size cuff. Given the arm circumference and height of an individual, the cuff may be selected which gives a value most closely approximating the intra-arterial systolic pressure.

is admittedly not precisely accurate. Moreover, one must consider the possibility that extraneously induced alterations in blood pressure may result from the mere introduction of the cannula into the lumen of the vessel. The former objection might have been eliminated had it been possible to devise a means of obtaining measurements at the same site, as well as at the same time. Needless to say, this was not possible.

The fact that all blood pressure determinations were made with the subject in a basal state, however, reduced the range of error which is introduced when comparative measurements are obtained asynchronously.

BLOOD PRESSURE MEASUREMENT
BY THE FLUSH TECHNIQUE

The determination of arterial pressure by auscultation has, until recent years, been the only method which is both sufficiently practical and accurate to permit its clinical use. In infants, however, this means of measurement is often difficult if not impossible to obtain, mainly because of the feebleness of the vascular sounds in the antecubital space. Recognition of the need for a clinically useful method of arterial pressure evaluation in the infant age group has resulted in a renewed interest in the flush method of measurement. This method has now been developed to such an extent that it is presently the one of choice for most infants under one or two years of age.

Technique

The procedure is best performed with the infant in a recumbent position. As with the auscultatory method, it is particularly important that he be quiet and relatively immobile since activity or crying may profoundly affect the readings obtained. To accomplish this end, it may be necessary to have the baby suck on a nipple or pacifier, even though the act of sucking may slightly increase the level of arterial pressure.

The arm cuff is applied to the wrist for an upper extremity reading and to the ankle for a lower extremity reading. The portion of the extremity distal to the cuff is then compressed by firmly wrapping it with a soft wide rubber drain beginning at the tips of the digits and working proximally to the lower edge of the cuff. In our experience, this is most readily accomplished when the dimensions of the elastic material are about 3-4 cm. in width and 50 cm. in length. When compression is completed, the cuff is rapidly inflated to 200 mm. Hg and the wrapping removed.

With gradual release of the manometer pressure, a level is reached at which there is a distinct flush of the blanched portion of the extremity. This is considered to be the end point (Fig. 7). Great care must be exerted not to release the pressure at a rate exceeding 5 mm. Hg per second and also to maintain the extremity at approximately the level of the heart. If the baby cries at any time during the measurement, the procedure should be re-

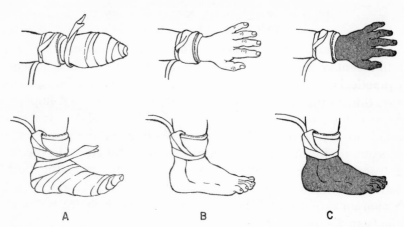

                    A   B   C

Fig. 7. Diagrams illustrating the technique of blood pressure measurement by the flush method. The cuff is applied to the wrist or ankle, and the distal portion of the extremity is wrapped snugly with an elastic bandage (A). The manometric pressure is then raised above the expected systolic pressure and the elastic wrapping removed (B). The blood pressure cuff is gradually deflated until the blanched portion flushes (C). This is read as the end point.

peated. In rare instances when accuracy is of particular importance, it may be necessary to sedate the infant.

Measurements should be made in a well-lighted room so that the visual acuity of the operator will be at a maximum. With practice, the first signs of the flush can be easily discerned. The degree of accuracy is probably increased when two observers work as a team to perform the measurement. One manipulates the compression bulb and reads the manometer while the other removes the elastic wrapping and observes the end point.

Width of the Cuff

According to our studies, the width of the cuff does not materially affect the readings obtained when measuring blood pressure by the flush technique.[43,44] A total of 118 infants were studied. In 68 of these, sequential flush measurements were made using a 5 cm. and a 7 cm. cuff and in 50, a 5 cm. and a 9.5 cm. cuff were used. The arithmetic means obtained in the first group were 71.50 mm. Hg for the 5 cm. cuff and 70.85 mm. Hg for

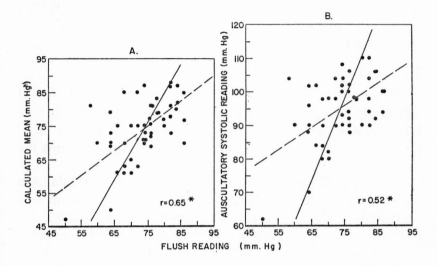

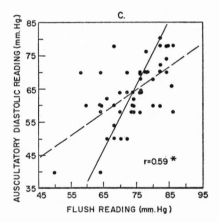

Fig. 8. Scattergrams illustrating (A) relationship of flush reading to calculated mean blood pressure, (B) relationship of flush reading to auscultatory systolic blood pressure, (C) relationship of flush reading to auscultatory diastolic blood pressure.

Broken line (- - -) indicates line of best fit when predicting auscultatory readings from flush readings.

Solid line (————) indicates line of best fit when predicting flush readings from auscultatory readings.

* r = Pearson Product - Moment Correlation.

the 7 cm. cuff. In the latter group, the arithmetic means were 68.08 mm. Hg for the 5 cm. cuff and 66.96 mm. Hg for the 9.5 cm. cuff. In neither case was the difference between the means considered to be significant.

Interpretation of the End Point

The end point of the flush method has been interpreted differently by different investigators. Whereas some[39,45,46] believe the earliest discernible flush represents the systolic level of blood pressure, our studies indicate that it more closely represents the mean pressure.

These studies comprised observations in 50 normal infants in whom the flush blood pressure was measured at the wrist and compared to the brachial auscultatory pressure obtained immediately thereafter using the same 5 cm. cuff.[43,44] The mean pressure was estimated by adding 1/3 of the pulse pressure to the brachial auscultatory diastolic pressure. It was found that the flush reading approximated the calculated mean pressure more closely than it did either the systolic or diastolic pressure. This relationship is graphically illustrated in Figure 8. The arithmetic mean of the auscultatory systolic values obtained in this study was 95.38, of the auscultatory diastolic values 63.88, of the mean values 74.56, and of the flush values 73.84 mm. Hg. A statistical test of the significance of the difference between these indicated that measurements by the flush method approximate to a greater degree the mean blood pressure than they do either the systolic or the diastolic auscultatory blood pressure (Tables III and IV).

The problem was further explored by making comparative studies of flush and intra-arterial measurements obtained in each

TABLE III

COMPARISON OF THE ARITHMETIC MEAN FLUSH PRESSURE TO THE ARITHMETIC MEAN OF THE AUSCULATORY SYSTOLIC, DIASTOLIC AND CALCULATED MEAN PRESSURES

	Systolic	*Diastolic*	*Flush*	*Calculated Mean Pressure*
Arithmetic mean	95.38	63.88	73.84	74.56
Standard deviation	10.28	9.36	8.03	9.24
Standard error of mean	1.47	1.34	1.14	1.32
Number of observations	50	50	50	50
Number of individuals	50	50	50	50

TABLE IV

SUMMARY OF STATISTICAL TEST OF DIFFERENCES BETWEEN THE ARITHMETIC
MEANS OF FLUSH AND AUSCULATORY BLOOD PRESSURES

	Mean Differences	*Standard Error of Mean Differences*	*"t" Test*
Flush versus auscultatory mean	0.72	1.12	0.65*
Flush versus systolic	21.54	3.44	6.26**
Flush versus diastolic	9.96	3.01	3.01**

* Not a significant difference.
** Significant difference at less than 1% level.

of a small group of subjects. A total of 17 observations were made
on 15 infants and children ranging in age from one hour to nine
years. Although the majority had some type of congenital heart
lesion, all but three were normotensive. The methodology for
this particular investigation was as follows:

In one subject, the infant who was one hour old, a No. 20
polyethylene tube 30 cm. in length was introduced into the
umbilical artery and advanced several cms. so that its tip pre-
sumably lay in the aorta. Pressures in this infant were measured
by a model P23A Statham strain gauge and recorded by a San-
born direct-writing recorder.

In all other subjects the studies were made under basal
anesthesia using 10 per cent Surital rectally (22 to 33 mg. per Kg.
body weight). In these a P23D Statham strain gauge was used,
and the pressure tracings were recorded by a direct writing Offner recorder. In some cases the direct measurements were made
through cardiac catheters inserted by way of defects into the
systemic circulation. In the majority, however, the femoral or
brachial artery was exposed and directly cannulated with a No.
20 needle after liberal perfusion with a 1 per cent solution of
Xylocaine. In seven subjects comparative flush measurements
were made in the contralateral extremity at the same heart beat.
In the subjects in whom central arterial blood pressures were
determined during cardiac catheterization, the flush measurements were made immediately after the catheterization procedure.

The natural frequency of the recording system when filled
with distilled water at 24°C. varied with the length and inner
diameter of the cannulating piece, but in no case was it below

TABLE V

DATA PERTAINING TO 17 OBSERVATIONS MADE ON 15 INFANTS AND CHILDREN IN WHOM DIRECT MEASUREMENTS OF ARTERIAL BLOOD PRESSURE WERE COMPARED TO READINGS OBTAINED BY THE FLUSH TECHNIQUE

Case No.	Age	Sex	Diagnosis	Site of Measurement	Direct Systolic Pressure	Direct Diastolic Pressure	Planimetric Mean Pressure	Flush Pressure
1	1 hr.	Female	Normal heart	No. 20 polyethylene tube in descending aorta	72	40	48	55
2	2 yr.	Female	Patent ductus	No. 6 cardiac catheter in descending aorta	96	60	72	80
3	4 yr.	Female	Tetralogy of Fallot	No. 7 cardiac catheter in ascending aorta	85	51	62	78
4	5 yr.	Male	Tetralogy of Fallot	No. 20 needle in femoral artery	116	70	93	86
				No. 8 cardiac catheter in ascending aorta	88	64	75	85
5	3 yr.	Female	Normal heart	No. 20 needle in femoral artery	116	70	93	86
6	11 mo.	Female	Tetralogy of Fallot	No. 6 cardiac catheter in ascending aorta	79	53	62	74
7	20 mo.	Male	Patent ductus and coarctation of aorta	No. 18 polyethylene tube in subclavian artery	145	60	88	126
				No. 7 cardiac catheter in descending aorta	45	23	28	50
8	2 yr.	Female	Interatrial septal defect	No. 20 needle in femoral artery	68	48	58	59
9	6 yr.	Female	Normal heart	No. 20 needle in femoral artery	98	64	76	66
10	5 yr.	Female	Patent ductus	No. 20 needle in femoral artery	104	58	68	70
11	7 yr.	Male	Subaortic stenosis	No. 20 needle in femoral artery	124	72	94	78
12	8 mo.	Female	Interatrial septal defect	No. 6 cardiac catheter in brachial artery	120	60	80	96
13	3 yr.	Male	Pulmonic stenosis	No. 20 needle in femoral artery	86	52	63	68
14	2 yr.	Male	Coarctation of aorta	No. 13 polyethylene tube in brachial artery	148	84	105	110
15	9 yr.	Male	Interventricular septal defect	No. 20 needle in femoral artery	104	74	86	82

With the exception of Case No. 14, in which a Lehman catheter was used, all cardiac catheters were of the Goodale-Lubin single lumen triple orifice type.

45 cycles per second. The mean blood pressures were calculated by planimetric integration of the pressure tracings.

The data pertinent to the study are presented in Table V. Because of the small sample of cases, a correlation study was statistically inappropriate. A statistical test, however, of the differences among the arithmetic means indicated that the flush values correlate more closely with the mean arterial pressure than with either the direct systolic or diastolic pressure (Table VI and VII).

TABLE VI

COMPARISONS OF THE ARITHMETIC MEAN FLUSH PRESSURE TO THE ARITHMETIC MEANS OBTAINED BY DIRECT ARTERIAL MEASUREMENTS

	Direct Systolic Pressure	Direct Diastolic Pressure	Planimetric Mean Pressure	Flush Pressure
Arithmetic mean	99.65	59.00	73.59	79.35
Standard deviation	27.05	14.23	19.30	19.07
Standard error of mean	6.57	3.45	4.68	4.63
Number of observations	17	17	17	17
Number of individuals	15	15	15	15

TABLE VII

SUMMARY OF STATISTICAL TEST OF DIFFERENCES BETWEEN ARITHMETIC MEANS BY FLUSH AND BY DIRECT ARTERIAL MEASUREMENTS

	Mean Differences	Standard Error of Mean Differences	"t" Test
Flush versus planimetric mean	5.76	3.18	1.81*
Flush versus systolic	20.29	3.33	6.09**
Flush versus diastolic	20.35	3.53	5.76**

* Not a significance difference.
** Significant difference at less than the 1% level.

Evidence presented by others supports the contention that the flush method of measurement more accurately reflects the mean than the systolic arterial pressure. Goldring and Wohltmann[47] had noted that flush values at the wrist were lower than auscultatory systolic values over the brachial artery but attached no special significance to their observation at that time. Earlier investigators[48-54] had found that the digital flush pressure was consistently and significantly lower than the brachial auscultatory systolic pressure. If the flush method were truly a measure of systolic arterial pressure, one would not expect the values to be lower at the wrist or finger than systolic readings obtained by auscultation over the brachial artery.[13,55-57]

Reliability of Results

The flush method of blood pressure measurement is now known to be sufficiently accurate for clinical use. This facet of the problem was resolved in a study by us in which measurements by the flush technique were obtained simultaneously in each of the upper extremities of 50 infants and in each of the lower extremities of an additional 50 infants.[43,44] Four observers participated in this study, each team of two members simultaneously recording measurements in the manner previously described. It must be confessed that although these readings were intended to be simultaneous, they were in effect sequential since it was impossible for the two teams to release the pressure in such a manner that the end points were reached at the same heart beat. However, the measurements were sufficiently close in time to eliminate for the most part such variables as might be ascribed to voluntary movements.

A correlation analysis of the paired observations revealed that the Pearson product-moment correlation coefficient was 0.87 for the lower extremity study and 0.65 for the upper extremity study. The smaller value for the upper extremity study may partially be explained by the greater incidence of intra-arterial blood pressure difference between the two upper limbs. The figures, nevertheless, indicate a high degree of reliability. This is further demonstrated in the scattergram shown in Figure 9.

OTHER INDIRECT METHODS OF MEASUREMENT

Of the many procedures for the indirect estimation of blood pressure, the auscultatory method for older children and the flush methods for infants are currently the most popular. Other methods include digital palpation and visual oscillometry — or instrumental modifications of these procedures. However, these

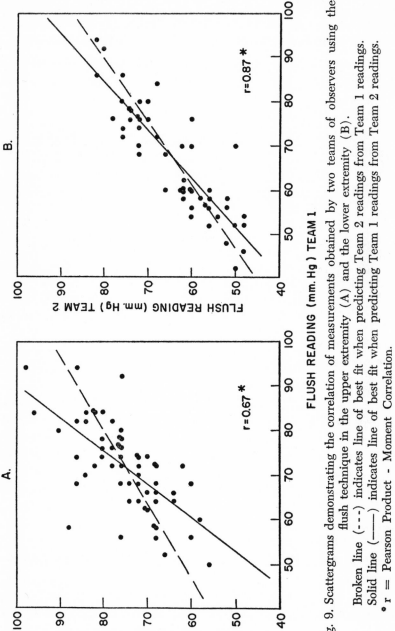

FLUSH READING (mm. Hg) TEAM 1

Fig. 9. Scattergrams demonstrating the correlation of measurements obtained by two teams of observers using the flush technique in the upper extremity (A) and the lower extremity (B).

Broken line (- - -) indicates line of best fit when predicting Team 2 readings from Team 1 readings.
Solid line (———) indicates line of best fit when predicting Team 1 readings from Team 2 readings.
* r = Pearson Product - Moment Correlation.

are generally either obsolete, too cumbersome for medical use, or not yet of proven value.

Digital Palpation

Estimation of the arterial pressure by palpation is the oldest of the clinically acceptable methods of indirect measurement. The method as it is used today is quite similar to that originally described by Riva-Rocci. The radial pulse is palpated, and the pressure in the arm cuff is raised to about 30 mm. Hg above the level at which the pulsations disappear. The system is then decompressed at a rate of about 2 to 3 mm. Hg per heart beat. The manometer pressure at the first palpable beat is recorded as the systolic pressure. The reading obtained by this method is usually 5-10 mm. Hg lower than that registered by auscultation.[38]

At one time estimation of blood pressure by this method was widely used in infants. Since the advent of the flush technique, however, measurement by palpation is used only when the flush or auscultatory methods are not feasible. In older subjects it may be of value in estimating the systolic pressure prior to measurement by auscultation.

Visual Oscillometry

The oscillatory or visual method of measuring blood pressure as it is practiced today was first introduced in 1904. It is based upon visualization of the oscillations which are transmitted by the arterial pulsations to the mercury column of the manometer.

The sphygmomanometer cuff is applied in the usual fashion and inflated to a level well beyond the expected systolic pressure. With gradual deflation, the levels at which the mercury oscillations appear and disappear are respectively read as the systolic and diastolic pressures.

Many modifications of this procedure have been introduced, and a number of oscillometers are now commercially available.[58,59] For the most part their use is restricted to investigational studies or to observations in adults with peripheral vascular disease.

Instrumental Palpation and Oscillography

Arterial pressure measurement by palpation or visual oscillometry may be modified so that the pulsations are recorded by various types of instruments. For this purpose a second sphygmomanometer cuff, or some other type of plethysmograph, is applied distal to the pressure cuff.[59] As the proximal cuff is slowly decompressed, the pulsations penetrate the arterial segment and are registered by the distal plethysmographic device.

When measurements are made by instrumental palpation, the pressure in the proximal cuff (pressure cuff) is recorded at the onset and cessation of the deflections registered by the distal recording device. As in digital palpation, these are believed to represent the systolic and diastolic pressure levels. When measurements are made by instrumental oscillography, the shape and size of the deflections rather than their appearance and disappearance are the criteria of measurement.

Shaffer[60] reported a study in newborn infants in which the pulsations distal to the occluding cuff were registered by impedance plethysmography. This procedure is based on the principle that impedance to a high frequency alternating current sent through a segment of the forearm changes with each arterial pulsation. The variations of impedance are detected by a bridge circuit and are recorded simultaneously with the pressure in the arm cuff on a twin channel recorder. In this way the systolic and diastolic levels of pressure can be determined. Shaffer's data indicate, however, that the diastolic pressure could not be measured with any degree of certainty.

More recently, Endres *et al.*[61] reported a similar study in which an electric microphone is applied to the extremity distal to the pressure cuff. The transmitted pulse waves are recorded on a single or multichannel electrocardiograph or on an oscilloscope. Their sample of comparative direct measurements was too small to attest to the accuracy of the method.

Morse and his co-workers[62] employing this same principle again, no studies were reported on the reliability of the method. attached the microphone directly to the blood pressure cuff. Here

SUMMARY

The optimal conditions for arterial pressure measurement cannot as yet be accurately defined. Whenever possible, efforts should be made to approach basal conditions by reassuring the child and allowing time for recovery from apprehension or recent activity.

The instrument itself is a frequent source of error. In selecting the manometer, a careful inspection for mechanical defects is an essential prerequisite.

For precise readings, certain precautions in technique must be observed. The mercury column should be vertical, and the observer's eye should be level with the meniscus. It is important also to select a cuff of appropriate width since one too narrow or too wide may give rise to error. The cuff should be inflated rapidly and deflated slowly — at the rate of about 5 mm. Hg per second.

The auscultatory method of arterial pressure measurement is applicable to all age groups with the exception of early infancy. The beginning of the first sound phase is taken as the index of the systolic pressure. The diastolic pressure is considered by some to be reflected by the muffling in sounds and by others by the disappearance of sounds. This remains a controversial issue.

The mechanism whereby the Korotkoff vascular sounds arise is still not clear. Throughout the years the explanations which have been proposed are: (1) sudden expansion of the vessel wall, (2) the "water hammer" phenomenon, (3) the "pre-anacrotic phenomenon," (4) the "Bernoulli effect," and (5) turbulence of blood flow.

Proper selection of the sphygmomanometer cuff is of great importance. Our studies indicate that the most important parameters for selection are arm circumference and body height.

The flush method is probably the method of choice in most infants under one or two years of age. The arm cuff is applied to the wrist or to the ankle, and the portion of the extremity distal to it is compressed with a soft, wide rubber drain. The cuff is then rapidly inflated to about 200 mm. Hg, and the elastic wrapping is removed. With gradual release of the manometer pressure, a flush appears in the hand or foot, and this is considered to be the end point. Whether the end point represents the systolic or mean arterial pressure has not been firmly established. Our studies suggest that it may represent the mean blood pressure.

Other indirect methods of measurement consist of digital palpation, of visual oscillometry, or of instrumental modifications of these procedures. For the most part these methods are obsolete, are too complex and cumbersome for general use, or are not yet of proven value.

REFERENCES

1. Allegretti, A. J.: Blood pressure as affected by altitude, *M. Bull. Veterans Admin., 19*:290, 1943.
2. Franke, K.: Neuere Anschauungen uber den Einfluss den Menschen, *Fortschr. Med., 50*:509, 1932.
3. Gottlieb, J. S.: Effect of changes in environmental temperature on blood pressure and pulse rate in normal men, *Am. J. Physiol., 113*:181, 1935.
4. Martinez Alvarez, A.: Studies of relationship between atmospheric phenomena and human physiology. *Puerto Rico J. Pub. Health & Trop. Med., 9*:210, 1933.
5. Rotta, A., and Miranda, A.: Normal values of the arterial pressure and frequency of arterial hypertension in high altitudes (abstract), *Am. Heart J., 37*:670, 1949.
6. Saile, F.: Uber den einflus der vegetarischen Ernahrung auf den Blutdruck, *Med. Klin, 26*:929, 1930.
7. Shilling, C. W., Hawkins, J. A., and Hansen, R. A.: Influence of increased barometric pressure on pulse rate and arterial blood pressure, *U. S. Nav. M. Bull., 34*:39, 1936.
8. Comstock, G. W.: Epidemiologic study of blood pressure levels in a biracial community in sourthern United States, *Am. J. Hyg., 65*:271, 1957.
9. Erlanger, J., and Hooker, D. R.: An experimental study of blood-pressure and of pulse-pressure in man, *Johns Hopkins Hosp. Rep., 12*:145, 1904.
10. Brooks, H., and Carroll, J. H.: A clinical study of the effects of sleep and rest on blood-pressure, *Arch. Int. Med., 10*:97, 1912.
11. Cotton, T. F., Rapport, D. L., and Lewis, T.: After effects of exercise on pulse rate and systolic blood pressure in cases of "Irritable Heart," *Heart, 6*:269, 1917.

12. Brigden, W., Howarth, S., and Sharpey-Schafer, E. P.: Postural changes in the peripheral blood-flow of normal subjects with observations on vasovagal fainting reactions as a result of tilting, the lordotic posture, pregnancy and spinal anaesthesia, *Clin. Sc.,* 9:79, 1950.

13. Kroeker, E. J., and Wood, E. H.: Comparison of simultaneously recorded central and peripheral arterial pressure pulses during rest, exercise, and tilted position in man, *Circulation,* 3:623, 1955.

14. Innes, G., Millar, W. M., Valentine, M.: Emotion and blood pressure, *J. Ment. Sc.,* 105:840, 1959.

15. Halliburton, W. D.: Traube waves and Mayer waves, *Quart. J. Exp. Physiol.,* 12:227, 1920.

16. Levine, S. A. and Harvey, W. P.: *Clinical Auscultation of the Heart,* Philadelphia and London, Saunders, 1949.

17. Ragan, C., and Bordley, J., III: Measurements of blood pressure, *Bull. Johns Hopkins Hosp.,* 69:526, 1941.

18. Bordley, J., III, Connor, C. A. R., Hamilton, W. F., Kerr, W. J., and Wiggers, C. J.: Recommendations for human blood pressure determinations by sphygmomanometers, *Circulation,* 4:503, 1951.

19. Bordley, J., III, Connor, C. A. R., Hamilton, W. F., Kerr, W. J., and Wiggers, C. J.: Recommendations for human blood pressure determinations by sphygmomanometers, *J.A.M.A.,* 147:632, 1951.

20. Burton, A. C.: Peripheral circulation, *Ann. Rev. Physiol.,* 15:213, 1953.

21. Korotkoff, N. S.: On methods of studying blood pressure, *Izviest. Imp. Voyenno-Med. Akad. S-Peterb.,* 11:365, 1905.

22. Rappaport, M.B., and Luisada, A. A.: Indirect syhygmomanometry, *J. Lab. & Clin. Med.,* 29:638, 1944.

23. Erlanger, J.: The movements of an artery within the compression chamber during indirect estimations of the blood pressure, *Am., J. Physiol.,* 39:401, 1916.

24. Erlanger, J.: Studies in blood pressure estimation by indirect methods, II, *Am. J. Physiol.,* 40:82, 1916.

25. Korns, M. H.: Nature and time relations of the compression sounds of Korotkoff in man, *Am. J. Physiol.,* 76:246, 1926.

26. Erlanger, J.: Relationship of longitudinal tension to the preanacrotic breaker phenomenon, *Am. Heart J.,* 19:398, 1940.

27. Erlanger, J.: Studies in blood pressure estimation by indirect methods, III, *Am. J. Physiol.,* 55:85, 1921.

28. Rodbard, S.: The significance of the intermediate Korotkoff sounds, *Circulation, 8*:600, 1953.
29. Lange, R. L., Carlisle, R. P., and Hecht, H. H.: Observations on vascular sounds: the "pistol-shot" sound and the Korotkoff sound, *Circulation, 13*:873, 1956.
30. Lange, R. L., and Hecht, H. H.: Genesis of pistol-shot and Korotkoff sounds, *Circulation, 18*: 975, 1958.
31. Malcolm, J. E.: *Blood Pressure Sounds and Their Meanings*, London, Heinemann, 1957.
32. von Recklinghausen, H.: Unblutige blutdruckmessung, *Arch. exper. Path. U. Pharmakol., 55*:375, 1906.
33. von Recklinghausen, H.: Neue wege der blutdruckmessung. Funf abhandlungen uber blutdruck und puls in den grossen arterien des menschen; zwei-messtellenvergleichmessung. Gleichheit des systolischen, verschiedenbeit des diastolischen drucks in den grossen arterien, *Ztschr. klin. Med., 113*:157, 1930.
34. Schaffer, A. I.: Neonatal blood pressure studies, *A.M.A. Am. J. Dis. Child., 89*:204, 1955.
35. Rushmer, R. F.: *Cardiac Diagnosis*. A physiologic approach, Philadelphia and London, Saunders, 1956.
36. Robinow, M., Hamilton, W. F., Woodbury, R. A., and Volpitto, P. P.: Accuracy of clinical determinations of blood pressure in children, *Am. J. Dis. Child., 58*:102, 1939.
37. Woodbury, R. A., Robinow, M., and Hamilton, W. F.: Blood pressure studies on infants, *Am. J. Physiol., 122*:472, 1938.
38. Guntheroth, W. G., and Nadas, A. S.: Blood pressure measurements in infants and children, *Ped. Clin. North America.*, Feb. 257, 1955.
39. Joos, H. A., Littlejohn, C. G., Bao, K. S., and Stanton, R. E.: Arterial blood pressure in infancy and childhood measured by direct and indirect methods, *Am. Soc. Ped.* Research Meetings, Swampscott, Mass., May, 1960.
40. Bazett, H. C., and Laplace, L. B.: Studies on indirect measurement of blood pressure; sources of error in Riva-Rocci method, *Am. J. Physiol., 103*:48, 1933.
41. Nuessle, W. F.: The importance of a tight blood pressure cuff, *Am. Heart J., 52*:905, 1956.
42. Wood, E. H.: Study of minimal dynamic response characteristics of manometer systems required for adequate recording of peripheral arterial pressure pulses in man. *Am. J. Physiol., 163*:762, 1950.

43. Moss, A. J., Liebling, W., Austin, W. O., and Adams, F. H.: An evaluation of the flush method for determining blood pressures in infants, *Pediatrics, 20*:53, 1957.

44. Moss, A. J., Liebling, W., Austin, W. O., and Adams, F. H.: Determining blood pressure in infants. Use of the flush technique, *Calif. Med., 87*:166, 1957.

45. Segal, S.: Personal Communication.

46. James, S.: Personal Communication.

47. Goldring, D., and Wohltmann, H.: Flush method for blood pressure determinations in newborn infants, *J. Pediat., 40*:285, 1952.

48. Weaver, J. C., and Bohr, D. F.: The digital blood pressure. I. Values in normal subjects, *Am. Heart J., 39*:413, 1950.

49. Cohn, A. E., and Lundsgaard, C.: A study of the blood pressure by the method of Gaertner, especially in patients suffering from fibrillation of the auricles, *J. Exper. Med., 27*:487, 1918.

50. Hayashi, T.: Vergleichende Blutdruckmessungen von gesunden und Kranken mit den Apparaten von Gaertner, Riva-Rocci, und Frey. Inaug. Dissert., Erlangen, 1901 (cited from reference 48).

51. Doleschal, M.: Vergleichende Untersuchungen des gaertner'schen tonometers mit dem von Basch'schen sphygmomanometer. Inaug. Dissert., Basel, 1900 (cited from Reference 48).

52. Oppenheimer, E. T., and Prinzmetal, M.: Role of the arteries in the peripheral resistance of hypertension and related states, *Arch. Int. Med., 60*:772, 1937.

53. Mendlowitz, M.: Some observations on clubbed fingers, *Clin. Sci., 3*:387, 1938.

54. Mendlowitz, M.: Measurements of blood flow and blood pressure in clubbed fingers, *J. Clin. Invest., 20*:113, 1941.

55. Hamilton, W. F., Woodbury, R. A., and Harper, H. T.: Physiologic relationships between intrathoracic, intraspinal and arterial pressures, *J.A.M.A., 107*:853, 1936.

56. Hamilton, W. F., and Dow, P.: An experimental study of the standing waves in the pulse propagated through the aorta, *Am. J. Physiol., 125*:48, 1939.

57. Wood, E. H., Fuller, J., and Clagett, O. T.: Intraluminal pressures recorded simultaneously from different arteries in man (abstract), *Am. J. Physiol., 167*:838, 1951.

58. Christensen, B. C.: Oscillometric Studies. On the change of sensitivity of the oscillometer at the different pressures, and on the in-

fluence of the state of contraction of the arterial wall on the oscillometric curve, *Acta Med. Scand., 120*:474, 1945.

59. Ejrup, B.: *Tonoscillography After Exercise.* A New Method for Early Diagnosis of Organic Arterial Disease Leading to Intermittent Claudication and for Differential Diagnosis of Organic and Functional Arterial Diseases with a Special Type of Apparatus Adapted to this Purpose, Stockholm, Svenska Tryckeriaktieholaget, 1948.

60. Schaffer, A. I.: Neonatal blood pressure studies, *A.M.A.J. Dis. Child., 89*:204, 1955.

61. Endres, R. K., Goldring, D. and Behrer, M. R.: Blood pressure studies in infants and children with an electric microphone, *J. Pediat., 52*:1, 1958.

62. Morse, R. L., Brownell, G. L., and Currens, J. H.: The blood pressure of newborn infants: Indirect determination by an automatic blood pressure recorder in 20 infants, *Pediatrics, 25*:50, 1960.

Chapter III

DIRECT BLOOD PRESSURE MEASUREMENT

Estimation of the arterial blood pressure by direct intra-arterial cannulation has long been useful in cardiovascular research. With the advent of cardiac catheterization and more recently of cardiac surgery, this method of measurement has come to play an important role in clinical medicine as well.

Currently, it is the method of choice whenever a continuous or a precise registration of the arterial pressure is required — a need which is encountered more and more frequently in the operating room, in the recovery room, and on the ward. The modern clinician, then, must understand not only the application and interpretation of this method of measurement but also the physical features and essential requirements of the necessary equipment.

TECHNIQUE OF ARTERIAL PUNCTURE

Although percutaneous puncture of a peripheral artery is commonly used in adults, our experience indicates that in infants and young children more accurate pressure tracings are obtained if the vessel is surgically exposed and cannulated under direct vision. In this way a No. 20 to No. 18 cannula can be inserted. Small bore bevelled needles generally used for percutaneous puncture are almost invariably occluded to some extent by the wall of the tiny vessel, and a significant degree of damping usually results. Moreover, in circumstances requiring prolonged registration of pressure, fixation of such a needle within the lumen of the vessel is less secure by the percutaneous method than with direct exposure.

It has been our practice to select either the femoral artery or the ulnar branch of the brachial artery. The skin is first rendered aseptic by scrubbing with Phisohex solution and then

44

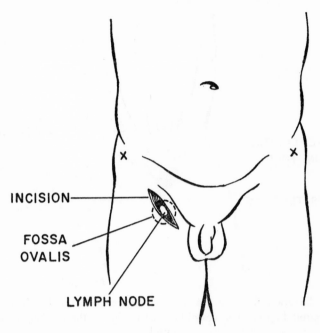

Fig. 10. Diagram illustrating the surgical approach to the femoral artery. The incision is made 1 cm. below the inguinal fold at a point where the arterial pulsations are maximal. The femoral artery lies posterior to the lymph node occupying the fossa ovalis.

rinsing with tincture of Zephiran. The field is surgically draped, and the area is infiltrated with a local anesthetic such as a 1 per cent solution of Xylocaine.

In the case of the femoral artery, a horizontal incision is made approximately 1 cm. below the inguinal crease at a point where the arterial pulsations are maximal. The subcutaneous tissues are divided by blunt dissection, and the lymph node occupying the fossa ovalis is exposed. Although there may be some individual variation, the femoral artery generally lies directly posterior to this structure (Fig. 10). Using the pulsations of the vessel as a guide, it usually can be readily exposed by blunt dissection.

In the case of the ulnar branch of the brachial artery, a horizontal skin incision is made approximately 1 cm. below the antecubital fold directly over the area of maximal arterial pulsa-

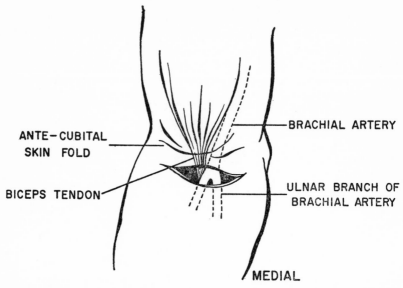

Fig. 11. Diagram showing the surgical approach to the brachial artery in the antecubital space. The vessel lies just medial to the tendon of the biceps muscle.

tions (Fig. 11). Using blunt dissection, the tendon of the biceps muscle is isolated and retracted to one side. With the pulsations as a guide, the vessel can generally be located with little difficulty.

When the artery is exposed, it should be perfused liberally with a 1 per cent solution of Xylocaine to inhibit vascular spasm. The vessel is then carefully stripped, and two ligatures are passed about it. An arterial cannula is inserted into the lumen of the vessel and secured in place with the proximal ligature. The obturator is withdrawn, and the cannula is connected to the manometer system.

Upon completion of the measurement, the cannula is removed, and the bleeding from the puncture site is controlled by firm pressure with a loose gauze. Five minutes of pressure is generally sufficient to stop the bleeding. In rare instances, particularly with prolonged observations, the vessel may become lacerated and repair with arterial silk may be necessary to control the bleeding.

FUNCTIONAL CHARACTERISTICS OF
THE MANOMETER SYSTEM

In order to study the details of a pulsatile pressure, the manometer system must be sufficiently sensitive to register the systolic and diastolic pressures as readily measurable deflections. The arterial pressure wave is a complex signal with a unique

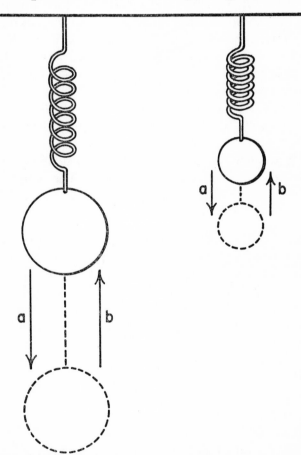

Fig. 12. The frequency response of a manometer is mainly determined by the ratio of the restoring forces to the inertia, just as for a weight suspended on a spring. The system on the left with its large mass and loose spring responds less quickly than the system on the right with its small mass and stiff spring. The length of the arrows (a and b) indicates how far each spring must be stretched to give the same restoring force.

harmonic content for a given wave. The function of the manometer system is to faithfully reproduce this signal. In addition
to *sensitivity,* this requires an adequate frequency response, as
well as a critical degree of damping.

The characteristic of a manometer system to react rapidly
enough to faithfully reproduce a fluctuating signal is referred
to in terms of *frequency response.* The higher the frequency
response, the more rapidly can the system follow changes in
pressure. The frequency response is expressed as vibrations or
cycles per second and is mainly determined by the ratio of the
restoring forces to the inertia. The greater the inertia, the less
will be the frequency response (Fig. 12). Thus, mercury with
its very high inertia in relation to the force of displacement and
restitution has a low frequency response and is not suitable for
the registration of arterial pressure pulses.

The frequency response of a system depends upon its natural
frequency and upon the degree of damping. The *natural frequency* may be defined as the "free" oscillations of the instrument

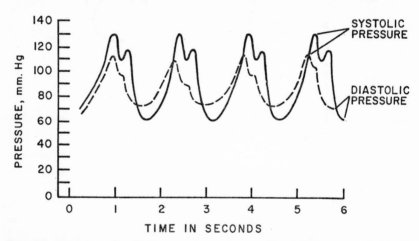

Fig. 13. Diagram showing a continuous recording of the arterial blood
pressure using a manometer system which is underdamped (solid line).
The oscillations arising from the manometer system itself are superimposed on the pressure pulse and cause elevation of the systolic peak and
depression of the diastolic dip ("overshoot"). The broken line represents
the recording which would have been obtained with an optimally damped
system.

itself. These instrumental oscillations when superimposed upon those of the signal cause a distortion of the pressure tracing and are therefore not desirable. The natural frequency of a manometer system may be partially overcome by damping.

Damping is the inhibiting effect which friction or other dissipative forces exert on oscillations. This effect is due to dissipation of a portion of the pressure energy in the form of frictional resistance. The longer the connecting tubes of the hydraulic system and the smaller their cross-sectional area, the greater is the frictional resistance and thus also the degree of damping.

If damping were completely absent, the system would have an undamped natural frequency. When a system is undamped or *underdamped,* the superimposed instrumental oscillations cause the diastolic pressure to be lower and the systolic pressure to be higher than their actual levels ("overshoot") (Fig. 13).

With *overdamping* the diastolic depression is higher and the systolic peak is lower than the actual levels. The waves are unusually smooth, and the upstroke is considerably delayed (Fig. 14).

Critical damping is the smallest amount of damping which will prevent the occurrence of instrumental oscillations. Critical

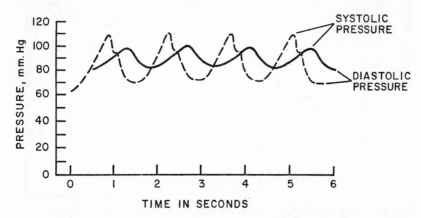

Fig. 14. Diagram showing a recording of the arterial pressure pulse using an overdamped manometer system (solid line). The waves are noticeably smooth, and the upstroke is delayed. The systolic peak is lowered, and the diastolic dip is raised. The broken line represents the recording which would have been obtained with an optimally damped system.

damping, however, is not necessarily *optimal damping* since the latter represents a compromise of the range of frequencies over which a uniform amplitude response is obtained and of the frequency response. The optimal degree of damping is considered to be about 70 per cent of critical damping.[1]

The frequency response of a recording system may be altered appreciably by a small drop of air contained within the fluid mass. This is because air is much more elastic than the diaphragm and acts in a sense as a "shock absorber." It is essential, then, at the beginning of each procedure to carefully examine the tubing and to eliminate all air bubbles by properly flushing the system.

It is essential also to check the linear and dynamic response of the recording apparatus at frequent intervals. The linear re-

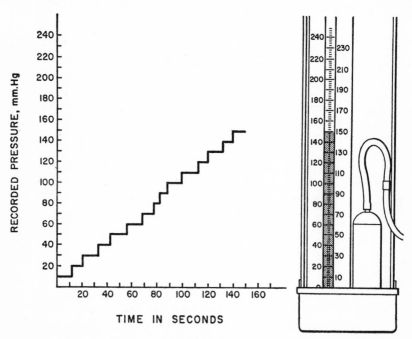

Fig. 15. Diagram of the record obtained when the linear response of a manometer system is checked. A mercury manometer is attached to the fluid end of the pressure system, and pressures are applied and recorded in "step fashion." The fidelity of the pressure apparatus is established by comparing the recorded values to those registered simultaneously on the mercury manometer.

sponse is determined by applying a known pressure, registered simultaneously on a mercury manometer, to the fluid end of the pressure system. The pressure is applied and recorded in "step-fashion" at increments of 10 mm. Hg over a wide range. At each level the fidelity of reproduction is established by comparing the recorded value to that registered on the mercury manometer (Fig. 15).

The dynamic response is determined by the so-called "square wave response."[2] This consists of the abrupt application and release of a momentary pressure to the fluid mass. The recorded deflection should closely approximate a wave of square dimensions (Fig. 16). A study of the characteristics of the recorded wave permits estimation of the degree of damping and of the frequency response of the system.

THE APPARATUS

The measuring and recording apparatus usually consists of an hydraulic system, a manometer, and a recorder. With electrical systems an amplifier is also frequently employed.

The Hydraulic System

This is represented by the fluid-containing connecting tubes which are attached to the intra-arterial cannula at the one end and to a diaphragm at the other. The diaphragm chamber and the tubes are filled with an anti-coagulant solution, the compressibility of which is negligible as compared to the displacement of the diaphragm. The enclosed fluid transmits the pressure waves from within the vessel to the diaphragm in the manometer.

The Manometer

This is essentially a diaphragm or membrane which is mechanically displaced by the pressure waves. There are two main types — mechanical and electrical.

Mechanical Manometers. These most commonly consist of a fluid-filled tambour with a diaphragmatic cover which is coupled to a recording lever. The frequency response in such a system is determined by the ratio of the weight of the lever and

THE DYNAMIC RESPONSE CHARACTERISTICS
OF PRESSURE RECORDING SYSTEMS

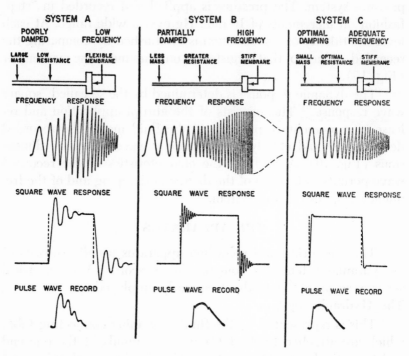

Fig. 16. The response characteristics of a recording system should be carefully established and rechecked frequently.

System *A* has a large mass of fluid in a large caliber tube and a flexible membrane. Thus, the system is very sensitive to changes in pressure but is poorly damped. If fluctuating pressures of constant amplitude and progressively increasing frequency are applied to the end of the tube, the output from the system increases with higher frequencies up to the natural frequency of the system and then declines. The characteristics of the system can be more easily checked by suddenly raising or abruptly lowering the pressure (a square wave of pressure). In this particular system, the recorded deflection was considerably delayed in reaching the new pressure level (slow rise time). The deflection had considerable overshoot and oscillations persisted at the natural frequency of the system for a considerable time (poor damping). This system would be entirely unreliable for recording arterial pressure pulses.

System *B* has a stiff membrane and partial damping. Pressure waves of equal amplitude produced a response of uniform height over a considerable range of frequency. However, the deflections became exaggerated near the natural frequency of the system. In response to a square wave, the rise time was very short and the oscillations at the natural frequency of the system died down rather promptly. This system would be adequate for recording pressure pulses unless certain portions of the pulse had frequencies near the natural frequency of the system. The square wave response should be determined just before using such a system because a single small air bubble in the catheter or the gauge may so reduce the response characteristics that system *B* acts like system *A*.

In system *C* the membrane is more flexible than that in system *B*, but system *C* has been critically damped. In other words, the output from the system is uniform throughout a wide range of frequencies. A square wave of pressure produced a rapid response and a very slight overshoot but no sustained oscillations. A critically damped system accurately reproduces arterial pressure pulses even though its uniform frequency response is limited to 20 or even 10 c.p.s. (Figure and legend from Rushmer, R.F.: *Cardiac Diagnosis; A Physiologic Approach,* Philadelphia and London, Saunders, 1956, p. 173.)

of the fluid contained within the system (inertia) to the flaccidity of the membrane (force of restitution) (Fig. 17).

The frequency response of a recording system is determined algebraically by the following equation:

$$N = \sqrt{\frac{E/M}{2\pi}}$$ where N = natural frequency, E = volume

elasticity of the system, and M = effective mass of the system. The effective mass is dependent upon the dimensions of the manometer and the weight of the enclosed fluid. This may be expressed as follows:

M = s L/Q where s = density of the solution in the manometer, L = length of the manometer, and Q = cross section of the liquid column.[3,4] It follows from the foregoing that the shorter and wider the liquid column and the more rigid the membrane, the greater will be the frequency response and the less will be the distortion of the recorded deflections.

If frequency response were the only determinant of fidelity, very effective mechanical manometers could be easily constructed. However, another quality of importance is the degree to which the magnitude of response is reproduced. This characteristic represents the *sensitivity* of the system. Sensitivity and frequency response oppose one another; i.e., the greater the

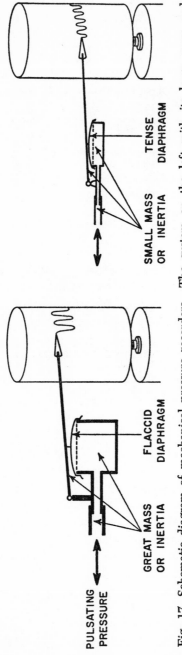

Fig. 17. Schematic diagram of mechanical pressure recorders. The system on the left with its large mass and flaccid membrane is very sensitive to slowly fluctuating pressures but will not reproduce rapid changes in pressure. The system on the right with its small mass and stiff membrane is less sensitive but has a greater frequency response. (After Rushmer, R. F.: *Cardiac Diagnosis; A Physiologic Approach,* Philadelphia and London, Saunders, 1956, p. 169.)

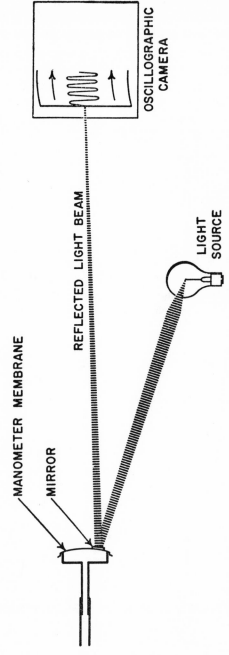

Fig. 18. Schematic diagram of an optical manometer. A beam of light is used in place of a lever to register the movements of a stiff membrane. Since light rays are weightless, great sensitivity is obtained without compromising the frequency response. (After Rushmer, R. F.: *Cardiac Diagnosis; A Physiologic Approach*, Philadelphia and London, Saunders, 1956, p. 169.)

sensitivity, the less the frequency response and vice versa. Efficient pulsatile recorders, then, must represent a compromise between sensitivity and frequency response in such a way that a maximum of sensitivity and a minimum of wave distortion are obtained (Fig. 17).

The efficiency of mechanical pressure manometers is considerably increased when an optical recorder is used. The latter consists essentially of a mirror which is mounted on the diaphragm in such a way that reflected light beams are diverted with displacement of the diaphragm. The optical deflections are registered by a recording camera (Fig. 18). Since light rays are weightless, the inertia due to the writing lever is completely eliminated and greater sensitivity is obtained without compromising the frequency response.

Utilizing this principle, Hamilton[5] and his associates developed a highly accurate optical system with a frequency response in excess of 150 cycles per second. He substituted a metal membrane of beryllium-copper for the rubber membrane. To compensate for the sensitivity lost because of the rigidity of the membrane, he devised an improved lighting system which magnified the deflections.

All mechanical manometers, however, including the high fidelity apparatus developed by Hamilton, have certain drawbacks which make their operation difficult. They are space consuming, difficult to fill with fluid, and their position must be firmly maintained while recording.

Electrical Manometers. Recent progress in the field of electronics has resulted in the development of a wide variety of electrical manometers. Because of their superiority in flexibility and perhaps also in fidelity of response, these have for the most part completely replaced the mechanical manometers. They are easy to fill, do not require rigid maintenance of position, and permit a wide range of alteration in the pressure and time scales.

With electrical manometers, the mechanical displacement of the diaphragm is converted to an electrical current which in turn may be amplified and recorded. The magnitude and time phase of the current is directly proportional to the degree of membrane displacement and therefore to the degree of applied pressure. Electrical manometers are therefore also *transducers* since in accomplishing the measurement, they must convert one form of energy into another.

The more common electrical manometers or transducers may be listed as follows:

A. Variable Resistance
   (1) Wire conductor
   (2) Carbon composition
   (3) Metallic film

B. Variable Reactance
   (1) Inductive
   (2) Capacitive

The *variable resistance* transducer consists of a conductive element which is either directly or indirectly attached to a diaphragm in such a manner that displacement of the diaphragm results in stretching or compressing the conductive medium. The latter is composed of wire, of carbon, or of a metallic film.

Electrical resistance may be defined as a measure of the resistance which a material object affords to the flow of an electric current. The resistance (R) of a circuit depends upon the length (L) or cross section (A) of the conducting medium depending upon the formula, $R = p L/A$, where p is the specific resistance of the material.

In the measurement of arterial pressure, the pressure waves are transmitted to the diaphragm by the hydraulic system, and the diaphragm is alternately displaced. The mechanical displacement in turn produces a variable strain on the conductive medium which is reflected proportionally by variations in electrical resistance (Fig. 19). These variations may then be amplified and recorded. Because the basic mechanism of the variable resistance transducer is the measurement of strain, it is commonly referred to as a *strain gauge*.

The variable reactance transducer may be either of the inductive or the capacitive type. As the terms imply, these are based upon the property of inductance or capacitance.

Inductance determines the electromagnetic force which is induced when a variable current flows through a wire. This force opposes the changes in the current and is therefore often referred

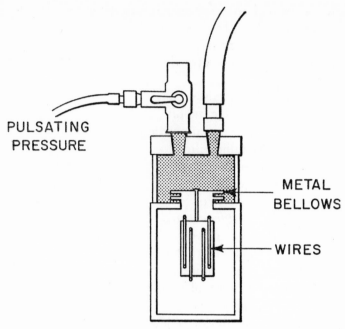

PULSATING
PRESSURE

METAL
BELLOWS

WIRES

Fig. 19. Diagram of an unbonded resistance wire strain gauge. The unbonded resistance wire strain gauge (Statham gauge) consists of a metal bellows which is compressed by increased pressure within the chamber. Downward displacement of the bellows is transmitted to a metal slide supported by four sets of strain-sensitive wires wound under tension and connected to form a Wheatstone bridge. Displacement of the metal slide stretches two sets of wires and relaxes the other two. These changes in resistance imbalance the bridge in proportion to the applied pressure. The resulting voltage output from the bridge is amplified and recorded by various means. (Figure and legend from Rushmer, R. F.: *Cardiac Diagnosis; A Physiologic Approach,* Philadelphia and London, Saunders, 1956, p. 171.)

to as the back electromagnetic force. It is extremely small for a straight wire, larger if the wire is coiled, and still larger if the wire is coiled around a soft iron core.

In the inductance type of transducer, a soft iron core is connected to the center of a diaphragm and the core is positioned within a system of wire coils. Displacement of the diaphragm by pressure from the hydraulic system causes movement of the iron core within the coils (Fig. 20). This produces an alteration in

APPLIED PRESSURE

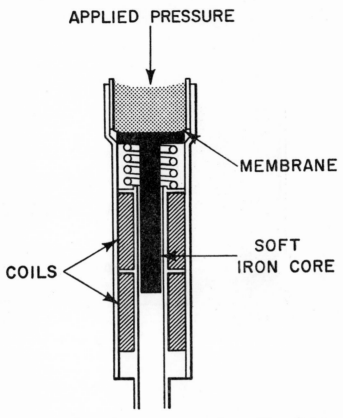

MEMBRANE

SOFT
IRON CORE

COILS

Fig. 20. Diagram of an inductance-type transducer. The soft iron core is connected to the membrane and is positioned within a system of wire coils. Displacement of the membrane results in movement of the iron core within the coils. The resulting alteration in inductance is reflected by an alteration in the level of the alternating current. (After Rushmer, R. F.: *Cardiac Diagnosis; A Physiologic Approach*, Philadelphia and London, Saunders, 1956, p. 171.)

inductance and therefore in the level of the alternating current. The pulsatile pressure of the blood when measured in this manner is reflected by fluctuations in the current which can then be amplified and recorded.

Capacitance is a measure of the capacity which a condenser has for storing an electric charge. A condenser consists of two metal plates which are separated by an insulator. The capacity

APPLIED PRESSURE

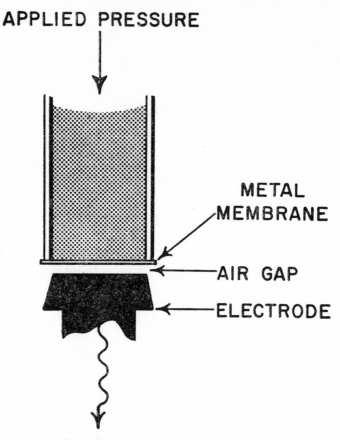

METAL
MEMBRANE

AIR GAP

ELECTRODE

Fig. 21. Diagram of an electrical capacitance diaphragm manometer. This is a condenser which consists of an electrode separated by an air gap from a stiff metal membrane. Movements of the membrane alters the thickness of the air gap and this causes a change in capacitance. (After Rushmer, R. F.: *Cardiac Diagnosis; A Physiologic Approach,* Philadelphia and London, Saunders, 1956, p. 171.)

of a condenser is determined by the size of the plates and by the extent of the separation between them. If they are relatively far apart, the capacity is small: if they are close together, the capacity is large. A variable condenser is one in which the capacity is altered by increasing or decreasing the distance separating the plates.

The capacitance transducer is a pressure gauge which has

as its basic mechanism a variable condenser. A stiff metal membrane in contact on one side with the hydraulic system is separated by an air gap on the opposite side from an electrode (Fig. 21). Displacements of the membrane due to fluctuations in pressure cause corresponding fluctuations in the capacity between the membrane and the electrode.

The Amplifier

Registration of blood pressure measurements require activation of a recording galvanometer. This is effected by the signal which is emitted from the electrical transducer.

Unbonded strain gauge pressure transducers produce a signal which is sufficiently strong without amplification to activate a photographically recording galvanometer. Such a system is stable and sensitive and entirely satisfactory in most respects. The one great disadvantage, however, is that once the recording has been started, it is difficult to alter the sensitivity of the system. This objection can be overcome if an amplifier is used.

With the other types of electrical transducers, the signal is so small that amplification is essential. When direct writing recorders are used, more extensive amplification is required because the inertia of the recorder is so great that the frequency response is limited. Even with the larger signal of the unbonded strain gauge, amplification is necessary if a direct writing recorder is used.

The Recorder

There are three basic types of recorders which are commonly used for the registration of blood pressure pulses:

     (1) Optical galvanometers
     (2) Direct writing galvanometers
     (3) Cathode ray oscilloscopes

Optical galvanometers make use of light beams which are amplified by an optical system and then deflected into an oscillograph camera. The most sensitive system consists of a galvanometer coupled to a resistance pressure transducer and an electronic amplifier. The flat frequency response of such a system is usually from 0 to over 100 cycles per second.

Objections to this type of recording device are that the

photographic process is tedious, and the record is not immediately available. Moreover, in the event the record is found to be defective, the entire procedure may have to be repeated.

Direct wiring recorders of several varieties are now commercially available. Their advantage in common is the provision of an instantaneous permanent record. The undesirable effect of pen inertia can be largely overcome by the use of compensating circuits so that the frequency response in some models is flat from 0 to 100 cycles per second.

Cathode ray oscilloscopes are vacuum tubes which contain an electric gun at one end, two pairs of deflector plates near the middle, and a fluorescent screen at the other end. The electron gun produces a narrow beam of high-speed electrons which are directed between the deflector plates. When they strike the flourescent screen, a luminous spot is produced (Fig. 22).

An alternating potential is applied to the deflector plates by the amplified signal, and this causes the electron beam to be deflected. The resulting pattern on the fluorescent screen may be observed directly or photographed.

Since the electron beam has negligible inertia, the frequency response of the cathode ray oscilloscope is practically unlimited.

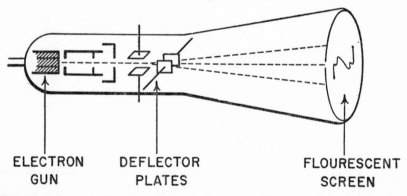

ELECTRON   DEFLECTOR   FLOURESCENT
   GUN   PLATES   SCREEN

Fig. 22. Schematic drawing of a cathode ray oscilloscope. The electron gun produces a narrow beam of high-speed electrons which pass between the deflector plates. When the beam strikes the fluorescent screen a luminous spot is produced. A voltage applied across the deflector plates causes the electron beam to be deflected and thus changes the position of the luminous spot.

It is generally of uniform amplitude (flat response) from zero to thousands of cycles per second.

THE ARTERIAL PRESSURE TRACING

Changes in the baseline (zero pressure line) may cause considerable error in the interpretation of pressure measurements. To insure accuracy, the baseline should be recorded before, during, and after each tracing since it may become unstable and drift at any time. The cause of drifting is usually attributable to changes in the temperature of the gauge.

The rate at which arterial pressure waves are customarily recorded is 25 mm. per second. However, most systems allow a variety of speeds, ranging usually from 10 to 100 mm. per second. The rate selected depends upon the purpose of the study. If the level of pressure is the primary interest, then a relatively slow speed is most satisfactory. If one is interested chiefly in the details of the pressure curve, then the deflections should be spread out by recording at a fast rate of speed.

The systolic pressure is represented by the very peak of the pressure wave and the diastolic by its low point. Since there may be a significant variation from heart beat to heart beat, the

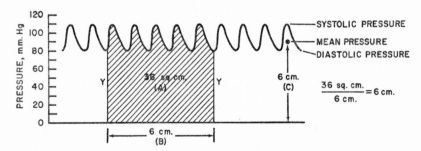

Fig. 23. Determination of the mean arterial pressure by planimetry. Since arterial pulse waves are not symmetrical, the arithmetic mean of the systolic and diastolic pressures does not represent the functional mean pressure. The latter is determined by measuring the area covered by several waves (shaded area A). This area divided by the horizontal dimension B gives the height of a rectangle which would occupy the same area. The quotient C represents the distance above the baseline where the mean pressure lies. (After Rushmer, R. F.: *Cardiac Diagnosis; A Physiologic Approach*, Philadelphia and London, Saunders, 1956, p. 168.)

average of a series of consecutive pressure wave measurements (at least five) should be taken to estimate the level of blood pressure.

The mean blood pressure is often used in calculating pulmonary and systemic resistances. It may be recorded directly by the use of integrating circuits which damp out the pulses, or it may be computed from the dynamic pressure curve by calculating the area under that curve. One standard method for accomplishing this is planimetric integration.

Planimetry is carried out by dropping vertical lines from each end of a series of pulse waves to the baseline. The area enclosed is measured by a special device called a planimeter, and the result is divided by the length of the baseline. The resulting quotient represents the distance above the baseline where the mean pressure lies (Fig. 23).

SUMMARY

Whenever a continuous or exact registration of blood pressure is required, direct intra-arterial measurement is the method of choice. In infants and children this is best accomplished by surgically exposing and then directly cannulating the femoral artery or a branch of the brachial artery.

The pressure waves are recorded by an apparatus whose component parts consist of an hydraulic system, a manometer, and a recorder. With most manometer systems, an amplifier is also used. Thorough familiarity with the physical features and requirements of the manometer equipment is essential, not only for the intelligent application of this method, but also for the appraisal of the results obtained.

The systolic pressure is represented by the very peak of the pressure wave and the diastolic by its low point. The mean blood pressure may be recorded directly, or it may be calculated from the dynamic pressure curve by planimetric integration.

REFERENCES

1. Noble, F. W.: *Electrical Methods of Blood Pressure Recording,* Springfield, Thomas, 1953.
2. Rushmer, R. F.: *Cardiac Diagnosis;* A Physiologic Approach, Philadelphia and London, Saunders, 1956.

3. Green, H. D.: Circulation: Physical Principles, Glasser, O. (Ed.):
   Medical Physics. Chicago, Year Book Publishers, 1944.
4. Green, H. D.: Circulatory System: Methods, Glasser, O. (Ed.):
   Medical Physics. Chicago, Year Book Publishers, 1950.
5. Hamilton, W. F., Brewer, G., and Brotman, I.: Pressure pulse contours in the intact animal. I. Analytical description of a new high-frequency hypodermic manometer with illustrative curves of simultaneous arterial and intracardiac pressures, *Am. J. Physiol., 107*: 427, 1934.

Chapter IV

BLOOD PRESSURE VALUES IN INFANTS AND CHILDREN

Estimation of blood pressure in infants and children can be accomplished by a variety of methods. Although a number of reports relating to arterial pressure measurements in the pediatric age group have appeared in the literature, variability of techniques and of methods used has precluded for the most part a clear-cut delineation between normal and abnormal values. The preliminary studies presented here were especially designed to overcome some of these objections. Nevertheless, considerable work remains to be done in this area.

For present purposes, the least complex approach to an analysis of the available data appears to be a consideration of the subject of arterial pressure values under three separate age categories; (1) in the neonate, (2) in the infant, and (3) in the preschool and school age child.

BLOOD PRESSURE VALUES IN THE NEONATE

Although information concerning blood pressure levels during the neonatal period has accumulated rapidly in recent years, the normal range of values has not yet been delineated. Much of the confusion stems from the fact that measurement by auscultation in this age group is not usually possible, and a suitable technique of measurement has not been established.

A wide variety of techniques have consequently been employed, and it is difficult to correlate the findings of one investigator using one method of measurement with those of another using a totally different method of measurement. Moreover, the sample size of most studies has been too modest to permit any definite conclusions.

A further factor is the width of the sphygmomanometer cuff. The effect of the width of the cuff within this age group has never been thoroughly investigated. How this might affect the blood pressure reading in the newly born infant has not yet been determined. The 2.5 cm. cuff has more or less arbitrarily been recommended for use in the neonatal period,[1-3] but we must agree with Schaffer[4] that this is probably too narrow.

A final difficulty in assessing the range of normal arterial pressure during this period is the present hiatus in our knowledge concerning the effect of the many normal and abnormal physiologic characteristics peculiar to the newborn — both before and after birth. A failure to consider these effects accounts in large measure for some of the conflicting reports in the literature.

Recent studies have demonstrated the importance of some of these influences. Ashworth and Neligan[5] found that the systolic blood pressure falls significantly during the first 24 hours of life. The rate of fall is affected by the clamping of the cord — a delay in clamping causing a delay in the rate of fall.

Neligan[6] observed that the systolic arterial pressure normally shows a propensity to drop from an initially high level. In infants delivered by caesarian section, however, this initial level is lower than in those delivered by the vaginal route. In premature infants with respiratory distress, the initial fall in arterial pressure is greater than in normal infants. Usher[6] found that in premature infants without distress the arterial pressure is lowest during the first 10 minutes of life and rises thereafter.

As in older subjects, the level of arterial pressure in the neonate is affected by sleep. Segal[6] observed that the pressure in the wakened but quiet and passive state is 10 to 15 mm. Hg higher than in the sleeping state.

Holland and Young[7] found that the systolic arterial pressure rises consistently during the neonatal period. With fetal anoxia and with abnormal forms of delivery such as cesarian section, it is significantly lower during the early post-natal period. They also found that the systolic pressure of premature infants was lower than in full-term infants and that this was directly related to the body weight. In a subsequent study[8] these same investigators demonstrated that during the first three to five days of life the systolic arterial pressure is not affected by tilting, whereas thereafter it is. They suggest that this may be due to some fundamental change in the circulation occurring at this time.

Woodbury and his co-workers[9] found that premature infants have low pressures which correspond to the length of gestation and that during the first 10 post-natal days, the brachial systolic pressure gradually increases. Forfar and Kibel[10] demonstrated that during the first 11 days of life the arterial pressure increases significantly with age and shows a positive correlation with birth weight.

The pressure existing within the umbilical arteries of newly-born infants has been studied extensively by James.[11] His conclusions reflect some of the general confusion regarding the range of normal for arterial pressure in the neonatal age group:

"It is difficult for me to give a meaningful figure which would accurately indicate the normal blood pressure in the new-born infant in the first hours after birth, since the range is considerable. The mean for our vigorous babies is 75/48 mm. Hg. However, for those in whom the cord is clamped immediately after birth, the mean is 69/43 mm. Hg with a range of 90/55 to 50/38 mm. Hg. In those where the placental blood was maximally given to the infant, the mean was 79/52 mm. Hg. In the depressed group of infants who were asphyxiated, some had higher blood pressures than average while others had lower, probably depending on the degree of asphyxiation and the vigor of resuscitation. The caesarian section group tended to have lower blood pressures than those delivered vaginally, but this was not invariable.

"In some instances we observed a fall in blood pressure over the first hour or two as did Neligan. These tended to be in more asphyxiated infants. In others there was little change in blood pressure over the first two or three hours.

"In summary, the range is considerable, and the measurement will be affected by the degree of asphyxiation, the mode of delivery and the volume of blood received by the baby from the placenta. Degree of maturity, I am sure, plays a role, but we have too few measurements to make any definitive statement about this."

It is clear from the foregoing that the problem of blood

pressure in the neonate is a complex one. Values are dependent upon the method of measurement employed, as well as upon factors related to fetal, natal and post-natal events. To date the range of normal has not been accurately defined. A brief tabulation of the data presently available for normal mature infants is given in Table VIII.

TABLE VIII

RANGE OF ARTERIAL BLOOD PRESSURE FOR NORMAL MATURE INFANTS

Investigator	No. of Subjects	Method Used	Average Blood Pressure (mm. Hg)
Woodbury et al[9]	24	Intra-Umbilical Artery (systolic and diastolic)	80/46
Holland and Young[7]	54	Palpation (systolic)	69
Neligan[6]	37	Plethysmograph (systolic)	56 - 84
Forfar and Kibel[10]	143	Flush (mean?)	74(arm) 82 (leg)
Ashworth and Neligan[5]	20	Plethysmograph (systolic)	60 - 92
Rice and Posener[12]	2	Plethysmograph (systolic)	77
Rice and Posener[12]	65	Flush (mean?)	65
Morse et al[13]	20	Modified Auscultatory (systolic and diastolic)	71/52
Moss et al[14]	145	Flush (mean?)	41 (arm) 37 (leg)

BLOOD PRESSURE VALUES IN THE INFANT

The determination of arterial pressure by auscultation in the small infant is extremely difficult because of the feeble vascular sounds. Consequently, the flush technique is the present method of choice for the estimation of arterial pressure in most infants. Preliminary studies which we conducted on a small scale[14,16] indicate that this is a measure of the mean rather than the systolic blood pressure, but there is no complete agreement on this point as yet.

Until recently, the normal standards for flush blood pressure values in infants were not known since reported measurements obtained from individuals with a normal cardiovascular status were too few to be statistically valid. The clinical need for such standards prompted us to conduct studies concerning this aspect of the problem.[14]

Observations were made on 551 normal Caucasian infants who ranged in age from one day to one year. At the time of each observation a complete physical examination was done. Only those subjects who had a normal cardiovascular status and who were free from acute and chronic infections were included in the study. The age, height, weight and the measurements of blood pressure by the flush technique in one upper and one lower extremity were recorded as a part of each examination. In all, 1712 flush readings were obtained—856 at the wrist and 856 at the ankle. All measurements were made in accordance with the technique previously described (see page 27).

The readings obtained were studied in relation to sex, body weight and age. The relationship of values in the upper to those in the lower extremity was also studied. Two types of analyses were made — cross-sectional and longitudinal. The cross-sectional study was comprised of one measurement selected at random from each of the subjects.

The ideal longitudinal study requires monthly measurements on every subject. These restrictions, however, would have reduced the available data to a handful of subjects for a very short range. A compromise was therefore attempted using the following restrictions: each subject must have had at least three measurements, the three or more measurements having been made so that approximately one month and not more than two months intervened between any pair of consecutive measurements. Under these restrictions 409 measurements were available from 105 individual subjects in 12 monthly age categories. Subjects for whom the measurements did not meet the restrictions for the longitudinal study were combined in the cross-sectional study with those for whom only one measurement was available.

The Relationship of Sex and Body Weight to Blood Pressure

There was no significant relationship between blood pressure and sex, nor between blood pressure and body weight within a given monthly age category during the first year of life. The supporting data are presented in Tables IX and X.

TABLE IX

MEDIANS OF THE BLOOD PRESSURE IN THE UPPER EXTREMITY OF THE
TWO SEXES IN EACH OF THE VARIOUS AGE GROUPS

Age (mo.)	No. of Male Subjects	Blood Pressure Median (mm. Hg)	No. of Female Subjects	Blood Pressure Median (mm. Hg)
1	24	61.6	27	61.7
2	35	69.0	15	65.0
3	31	68.8	25	69.0
4	21	72.6	17	74.0
5	18	73.0	10	73.0
6	20	70.2	28	71.5
7	14	77.5	10	73.0
8	13	79.0	10	77.0
9	15	80.0	16	76.0
10	16	74.0	6	79.0
11	10	73.0	5	73.0
12	12	76.0	8	77.0

It will be noted that within the same age category the median blood pressures
for males and females differ by at most 5 mm. Hg. These differences are not
statistically significant.

TABLE X

ø COEFFICIENT AND PROBABILITY VALUES RELATED TO BLOOD PRESSURE IN THE
UPPER EXTREMITY AND BODY WEIGHT WITHIN MONTHLY AGE CATEGORIES
*(The figures clearly indicate that the differences obtained are not significant
and therefore it is reasonable to assume that the body weight within a
given age category does not crucially affect blood pressure)*

Age (mo.)	No. of Male Subjects	ø Coefficient*	p**	No. of Female Subjects	ø Coefficient*	p**
1	24	0		27	+.26	.20>p>.10
2	35	+.03	.98>p>.95	15	+.05	.90>p>.80
3	31	−.17	.50>p>.30	25	−.04	.90>p>.80
4	21	−.30	.70>p>.50	17	0	
5	18	+.11	.70>p>.50	10	0	
6	20	0		28	+.07	.80>p>.70
7	14	+.14	.70>p>.50	10	0	
8	13	0		10	0	
9	15	+.06	.90>p>.80	16	0	
10	16	−.16	.70>p>.50	6	0	
11	10	0		5	0	
12	12	−.34	.30>p>.20	8	0	

** p = probability of ø.

* ø Coefficient $=\sqrt{x^2/N}$ and is an estimate of the Pearson product-moment
r coefficient of correlation.

The Relationship of Age to Blood Pressure

Blood pressure as related to age is demonstrated in Figure 24. This is based on measurements obtained on 551 infants. It will be noted that the arithmetic mean blood pressure shows a pronounced and highly significant rise after the first week of life. This is further illustrated by the numerical tabulation of

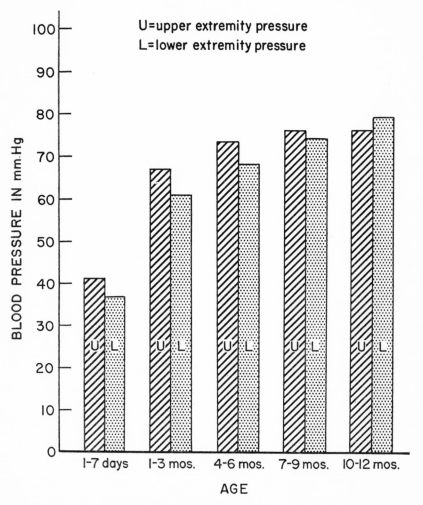

Fig. 24. Bar graph representing relationship of the arithmetic mean blood pressure and age in a cross-sectional study of 551 infants.

TABLE XI

Arithmetic Mean Blood Pressure (mm/Hg) in the Various Age Categories with Observed Range of Values and Predicted Range of Normal Expressed as ± 2 Standard Deviations

Age	No. of Subjects	Mean Blood Pressure at Wrist	Standard Deviation	Predicted Range of Values	Observed Range of Values	Mean Blood Pressure at Ankle	Standard Deviation	Predicted Range of Values	Observed Range of Values
1-7 days	145	41	±8	25-57	22-66	37	±7	23-51	20-58
1-3 mo.	155	67	±11	45-89	48-90	61	±10.5	40-82	38-96
4-6 mo.	115	73	±9.5	54-92	42-100	68	±10	48-88	40-104
7-9 mo.	79	76	±9	58-94	52-96	74	±8.5	57-91	50-96
10-12 mo.	57	76	±14	62-90	62-94	79	±8.5	62-96	56-102
1-12 mo.	406	72	±10.5	51-93	22-100	68	±12	44-92	20-104

the arithmetic means and the standard deviations for the first
week of life and for quarterly periods of the first year which are
presented in Table XI. From this data it cannot be stated whether
the rise after the first week of life is an abrupt or a gradual one.

Results of the longitudinal study conducted in 105 infants
are presented in Figure 25. The curve is based on monthly arithmetic mean blood pressures obtained during the first year of

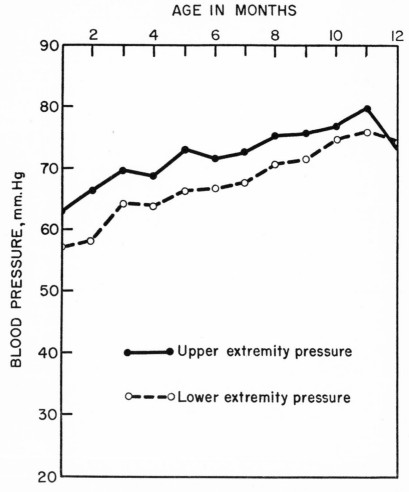

Fig. 25. Curve representing relationship between arithmetic mean blood
pressure and age in a longitudinal study of 105 infants.

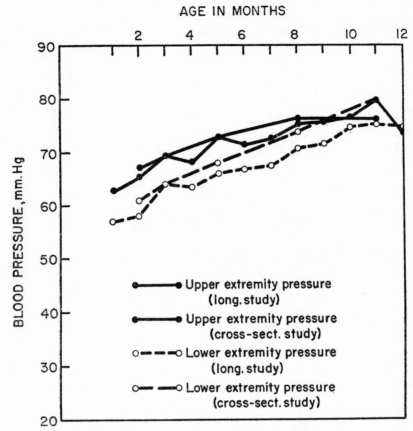

Fig. 26. Curve showing correlation between the longitudinal and cross-sectional studies.

life. The similarity of this curve to that in Figure 24 is best illustrated by the composite shown in Figure 26.

Assuming that ±2 standard deviations constitute the normal limits for flush blood pressures in infants, the range during the first year of life was found to be from 51 to 93 mm. Hg for the upper extremity and from 44 to 92 mm. Hg for the lower extremity. These figures are exclusive of the first week of life.

The Relationship of Blood Pressure in Upper and Lower Extremity

Reported observations have established that flush readings

obtained in the upper extremity differ from those in the lower extremity.[10,14,16,17] The extent and direction of this difference is, of course, extremely important when considering the diagnosis of coarctation of the aorta.

It is known that during the first nine months of life readings obtained at the wrist are somewhat higher than those at the ankle. Thereafter the converse is true. This relationship is apparent in Figure 24 but is perhaps better visualized in Figure 27. It will be noted that the first significant drop in the difference between pressure in the upper and lower extremity occurs between the sixth and seventh months of life. The process is completed and evidenced in a second significant fall between the ninth and tenth months, and thereafter the pressure at the ankle continues to exceed that at the wrist.

It is noteworthy that the initial trend for the reversal towards the adult pattern corresponds roughly to the age of sitting

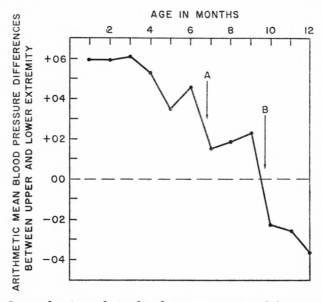

Fig. 27. Curve showing relationship between upper and lower extremity arithmetic mean blood pressure differences and age in a cross-sectional study of 406 infants. The initial trend toward reversal occurs between the sixth and seventh months (A) and is complete between the ninth and tenth months of life (B).

up and becomes complete at about the age of creeping. It is possible that the direction of the blood pressure gradient between the upper and lower extremity is related to the stage of motor development of the infant, particularly as it concerns posture and locomotion.

The blood pressure gradient between the upper and lower extremity in a given infant can be readily established by using an ingenious sphygmomanometer arrangement designed by Adams and his associates[18] for diagnosis of coarctation of the aorta. This consists of two cuffs (one for the wrist and one for the ankle) which are connected by one Y tube to a single manometer and by another Y tube to a single inflation bulb (Fig. 28). In this way the pressure in both cuffs can be measured simultaneously and intrinsic and extrinsic errors are largely eliminated, even if the subject is active or crying.

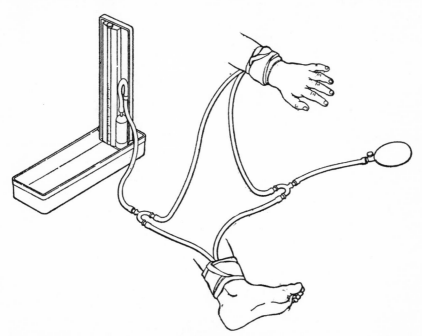

Fig. 28. Diagram showing the sphygmomanometer apparatus for simultaneous measurement of the flush blood pressure in the upper and lower extremities. The arrangement is of value in the diagnosis of coarctation of the aorta.

BLOOD PRESSURE VALUES IN THE PRE-SCHOOL
AND SCHOOL AGE CHILD

Beyond two years of age, measurement of blood pressure is best accomplished by the auscultatory method. However, in the past, estimations obtained by this method have had limited meaning because the range of normal values in children had never been fully established.

The principal objection raised to the data recorded in the literature was that cuff selection was, for the most part, based upon purely arbitrary means. In an effort to resolve this problem, we recently conducted a study aimed at establishing values which were believed to be minimally distorted by the effect of cuff size. The results obtained were found to be in surprisingly close agreement with those adapted from the literature by Haggerty and co-workers[19] and by Guntheroth and Nadas.[20]

Blood pressure measurements were made by us on a total of 1022 children ranging in age from 2 to 18 years. Each subject was determined to be in good health by previous examination. The appropriate cuffs were selected with the aid of the graph shown in Figure 6. In each case, the systolic pressure was recorded as the beginning of the first vascular sound phase and the diastolic pressure as both the point of muffling and the point of cessation. The systolic readings were adjusted according to the arm circumference and the height of the individual (Fig. 5). The adjusted value was believed to be the best estimate of the systolic blood pressure within the brachial artery. Because of previously demonstrated inaccuracies, the diastolic pressure reading was not accepted as a true value.

The Relationship of Sex to Blood Pressure

As with the flush method, no over-all relationship was found between sex and systolic arterial pressure (Table XII). However, within certain age categories there did appear to be a definite relationship to sex. This will be further amplified under the subsection concerned with age and blood pressure.

The Relationship of Age to Blood Pressure

The arterial blood pressure by sex and by age is presented in Tables XIII and XIV. It is to be noted that the systolic press-

TABLE XII

MEAN SYSTOLIC AND DIASTOLIC AUSCULATORY BLOOD PRESSURE
IN THE TWO SEXES

Sex	N	Adj Systolic		Diastolic 1		Diastolic 2	
		Mean	2 St. Dev.*	Mean	2 St. Dev.	Mean	2 St. Dev.
Male	(716)	110.1	21.2	67.8	28.6	48.9	43.6
Female	(306)	109.0	21.2	67.7	25.8	52.5	41.6

* Two standard deviations probably constitute the limits of normal for systolic
pressure.

ure in boys shows almost a uniform increase with age, whereas
in girls the peak pressure is reached at 12 years of age and thereafter declines.

TABLE XIII

THE RELATIONSHIP OF AUSCULATORY BLOOD PRESSURE TO AGE IN FEMALES

Age in Years	Adj. Syst. Mean	Stan. Dev.	Diast. 1 Mean	Stan. Dev.*	Diast. 2 Mean	Stan. Dev.*	N
< 2.50	98.0	9.2	60.0	11.1	26.7	23.2	3
2.50 - 3.49	93.6	5.4	63.6	12.9	38.8	22.7	5
3.50 - 4.49	99.3	8.4	66.0	9.8	46.6	14.9	17
4.50 - 5.49	99.2	5.9	62.2	8.9	39.0	16.4	10
5.50 - 6.49	103.2	5.6	63.5	8.9	37.2	20.6	16
6.50 - 7.49	108.0	7.0	73.1	8.8	50.9	17.1	9
7.50 - 8.49	105.1	8.9	68.7	10.6	42.9	28.5	14
8.50 - 9.49	108.0	9.1	68.0	16.2	53.5	23.5	42
9.50 - 10.49	108.3	7.0	71.3	8.7	60.5	11.0	49
10.50 - 11.49	114.0	11.2	67.1	16.4	56.5	22.1	51
11.50 - 12.49	117.1	10.9	67.0	15.0	55.4	15.9	45
12.50 - 13.49	112.0	7.2	65.5	9.0	41.4	25.3	19
13.50 - 14.49	108.9	14.1	63.7	12.4	52.9	23.2	7
14.50 - 15.49	104.8	7.2	75.2	8.6	67.6	11.3	5
15.50 - 16.49	106.9	10.2	72.9	10.6	61.8	19.2	9
16.50 - 17.49	106.0	19.8	60.0	14.1	51.0	21.2	2
17.50 - 18.49	96.0	11.3	68.0	11.3	66.0	14.1	2

305 Total

Diast. 1 = muffling of sounds.
Diast. 2 = cessation of sounds.
* Two standard deviations are considered as the limits of normal for systolic
pressure.

It is of considerable interest that this age trend of blood
pressure is almost exactly duplicated by that of cardiac response
to graded exercise tests in the two sexes.[21] It hardly seems likely
that this could be attributed solely to coincidence. However,
further studies are necessary before any real importance can be
attached to this observation.

TABLE XIV

THE RELATIONSHIP OF AUSCULATORY BLOOD PRESSURE TO AGE IN MALES

Age in Years	Adj. Syst. Mean	Stan. Dev.*	Diast. 1 Mean	Stan. Dev.*	Diast. 2 Mean	Stan. Dev.*	N
2.50 - 3.49	97.4	8.8	65.1	9.0	43.7	20.0	7
3.50 - 4.49	100.2	10.0	57.4	23.0	37.0	22.1	10
4.50 - 5.49	102.3	6.1	61.3	10.1	41.3	18.5	20
5.50 - 6.49	106.1	7.1	68.2	9.8	49.0	14.8	22
6.50 - 7.49	106.2	6.4	70.2	7.7	50.3	15.2	12
7.50 - 8.49	108.2	10.5	68.0	7.2	47.0	11.8	26
8.50 - 9.49	108.0	9.3	65.7	8.1	48.1	16.2	31
9.50 - 10.49	107.8	9.2	69.1	10.2	55.0	16.2	30
10.50 - 11.49	108.7	13.0	64.7	16.7	48.2	22.9	76
11.50 - 12.49	111.3	11.5	67.9	15.0	49.0	22.7	189
12.50 - 13.49	112.0	8.8	67.5	15.9	47.5	23.5	166
13.50 - 14.49	112.2	10.7	70.4	14.4	51.0	24.0	69
14.50 - 15.49	109.9	7.7	69.0	9.5	48.2	22.9	27
15.50 - 16.49	110.8	11.5	75.2	9.5	59.2	21.2	18
16.50 - 17.49	115.7	9.4	79.2	11.9	62.4	14.3	10
17.50 - 18.49	125.0	7.1	82.0	17.0	67.0	4.2	2

715 Total

Diast. 1 = muffling of sounds.
Diast. 2 = cessation of sounds.
* Two standard deviations are considered as the limits of normal for systolic pressure.

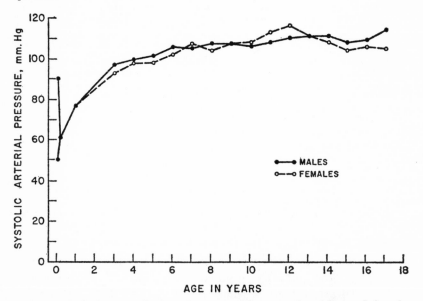

Fig. 29. Curve showing the systolic arterial pressure in males and females from birth to 17 years of age. The pressure increases steadily after the neonatal period until the age of puberty. It reaches its maximum in females at about 12 years and in males at about 17 years of age.

SUMMARY

The normal range of blood pressure is considered under three age categories: (1) in the neonate, (2) in the infant, and (3) in the pre-school and school age child.

In the neonate the techniques of measurement are so varied and the studies are so limited in number that, as yet, no limits of normal can be defined.

In the infant age group beyond the neonatal period, the flush method of measurement is probably the method of choice. Measurements made using this technique probably approximate the mean rather than the systolic blood pressure. Measurements of blood pressure show a pronounced and highly significant rise following the first week of life. During the first nine months of life the reading is somewhat higher at the wrist than at the ankle. Thereafter the converse is true. Exclusive of the first week of life, the range of normal blood pressure during the first year as determined by the flush method is from 51 to 93 mm. Hg for the upper extremity and from 44 to 92 mm. Hg for the lower extremity.

Beyond the ages of infancy, measurement of blood pressure is best accomplished by the auscultatory method. The systolic blood pressure in boys shows almost a uniform increase from two years of age to 17 years of age. In girls the peak systolic pressure is reached at 12 years of age following which there is a decline. For the entire age span, however, there is no significant difference in values for the two sexes. The mean systolic pressure (corrected for cuff error) is 110 mm. Hg in boys and 109 mm. Hg in girls.

REFERENCES

1. Bordley, J. III, Connor, C.A.R., Hamilton, W.F., Kerr, W.J., and Wiggers, C.J.: Recommendations for human blood pressure determinations by sphygmomanometers, *Circulation, 4*:503, 1951.

2. Robinow, M., Hamilton, W. F., Woodbury, R.A., and Volpitto, P. P.: Accuracy of clinical determinations of blood pressure in children, with values under normal and abnormal conditions, *Am. J. Dis. Child., 58*:102, 1939.

3. Day, R.: Blood pressure determination in children: Effect of width of cuff, *J. Pediat., 14*:148, 1939.

4. Schaffer, A. I.: Neonatal blood pressure studies, *A.M.A. J. Dis. Child., 89*:204, 1955.

5. Ashworth, A. M., and Neligan, G. A.: Changes in the systolic blood pressure of normal babies during the first twenty-four hours of life, *Lancet, 1*:804, 1959.

6. Neligan, G.: The systolic blood pressure in neonatal asphyxia and the respiratory distress syndrome, *A.M.A. J. Dis. Child., 98*:460, 1959.

7. Holland, W. W., and Young, I. M.: Neonatal blood pressure in relation to maturity, mode of delivery, and condition at birth, *Brit. M. J., 2*:1331, 1956.

8. Young, I. M., and Holland, W. W.: Some physiological responses of neonatal arterial blood pressure and pluse rate, *Brit. M. J., 2*: 276, 1958

9. Woodbury, R. A., Robinow, M., and Hamilton, W. F.: Blood pressure studies on infants, *Am. J. Physiol., 122*:472, 1958.

10. Forfar, J. O., and Kibel, M. A.: Blood pressure in the newborn estimated by the flush method, *Arch. Dis. Child., 31*:126, 1956.

11. James, L. S.: Personal Communication.

12. Rice, H. V., and Posener, L. J.: A practical method for the measurement of systolic blood pressure of infants, *Pediatrics, 23*:854, 1959.

13. Morse, R. L., Brownell, G. L., and Currens, J. H.: The blood pressure of normal infants: indirect determination by an automatic blood pressure recorder in 20 infants, *Pediatrics, 25*:50, 1960.

14. Moss, A. J., Liebling, W., and Adams, F. H.: The flush method for determining blood pressures in infants II. Normal values during the first year of life, *Pediatrics, 21*:950, 1958.

15. Moss, A. J., Liebling, W., and Adams, F. H.: The flush technique for determining blood pressure in infants. *California Med., 87*:166, 1957.

16. Goldring, D., and Wohltmann, H.: Flush method for blood pressure determinations in newborn infants. *J. Pediat., 40*:285, 1952.

17. Reinhold, J., and Pym. M.: The determination of blood pressure in infants by the flush method. Arch. Dis. *Childhood, 30*:127, 1955.

18. Adams, P. M., Keele, M., and Baronofsky, I.: Coarctation of the aorta in infants. *Essays on Pediatrics in Honor of Irvine McQuarrie,* Minneapolis, Lancet Publications, 1955.

19. Haggerty, R. J., Maroney, M. W., and Nadas, A. S.: Essential hypertension in infancy and childhood; differential diagnosis and therapy, *A.M.A.J. Dis. Child., 92*:535, 1956.

20. Guntheroth, W. G., and Nadas, A. S.: Blood pressure measurements in infants and children. *Ped. Clin.* North America, 257, Feb., 1955.

21. Adams, F. H., Linde, L. M. and Miyake, H.: The physical working capacity of normal school children: I. California. Accepted for publication in *Pediatrics*.

Chapter V

PHYSIOLOGIC INTERPRETATIONS OF AVAILABLE DATA

It is a common misconception that the arterial pressure rises uniformly from birth to old age. The data presented in the preceding chapter clearly indicate that this is not the case. The immediate post-natal period is characterized by a wide range of values and is followed by either a rise or fall in pressure in a given infant. Beyond the early neonatal period, the systolic arterial pressure increases steadily until the age of puberty, reaching its maximum in females at about 12 years and in males at about 17 years of age (Fig. 29). This pattern has been reported by others also.[1,2] The sharp divergence between the two sexes at puberty suggests the possibility that the process of sexual maturation either directly or indirectly affects the level of the systolic pressure.

Interest in the physiologic aspects of the arterial pressure in the young was first aroused in 1932 when Clark[3] obtained arterial pressure tracings on the embryo of a cat. It was subsequently shown that the arterial pressure increases with age in a variety of animals, as well as in man. This has been demonstrated in chickens,[4-6] turkeys,[7] sheep,[8] and rabbits.[9] The adult level varies with the particular species — being reached in weeks or months in some animals and in years in others. Contrary to the preceding observations, the systolic arterial pressure in the duck and in the pigeon has been reported to remain unchanged with increasing age.[10] This latter study serves to emphasize the potential hazard of extrapolating data from one species to another.

Interest in the arterial blood pressure of the young has extended down even into the life of the fetus. The systolic arterial pressure is now known to increase with fetal growth.

This has been observed in man,[11] in rats,[12] in sheep,[13-15] and in goats.[16]

The physiologic basis for these observations is by no means clear. It is not yet known whether the behavior of arterial pressure at a given age is the result of alteration in the cardiac output, the peripheral vascular resistance or both. On the basis of the evidence at hand, it might be postulated that changes in both cardiac output and peripheral vascular resistance are responsible for the early post-natal observations. Beyond this period the weight of available evidence suggests that an increase in cardiac output is the principal cause of the rising arterial pressure.

It has long been recognized that the total blood volume at birth is in large part determined by factors incident to delivery — particularly upon the interval between delivery and the clamping of the cord. This being the case, it may be assumed that cardiac output probably shows considerable variation from infant to infant at birth.

The central nervous system of the infant before, during and after delivery is subject to a variety of chemical, mechanical and thermal stimuli. Since these vary both in number and degree from infant to infant, it is likely that alteration in the peripheral vascular resistance mediated by the vasomotor reflexes play an important role in the observed differences of arterial pressure. Whether these reflexes are present in the human at birth, however, is still a moot question. The weight of available evidence suggests that in most animals the vasomotor reflexes are present and are functional at birth.

Studies performed by Clark[3] in 1932 indicate that in the cat the response of the fetal vasomotor center increases toward the end of pregnancy. Further studies on cats and dogs conducted in 1934, however, showed that although the vagus responds to artificial stimulation, the pathways are not active until after birth.[17] The cardio-aortic and cartoid sinus reflexes were believed to develop at four to six days after birth in puppies and at about 11 days in kittens. In the goat, Barcroft[16] demonstrated that vagal activity was, in part, responsible for the slowing of the fetal heart rate which occurred when the umbilical cord was occluded. It was later determined in sheep (1937) that the activity of the vagus was dependent upon the state of gestation.[18] In the 88 day sheep fetus the vagi were not involved in the fall of heart rate coincident with clamping of the cord, but in the 119 day fetus they were. Shortly afterward (1939), Bauer[9,19] found that the depressor and carotid sinus reflexes could be elicited in the rabbit at 11 to 14 days after birth but did not appear under ordinary conditions until about 40 days for the depressor reflex and about 50 days for the carotid sinus reflex. He could not demonstrate that the vagal pathways were functional in the rabbit in utero.

These earlier studies indicate that vagal action differs in different animals. It has been postulated that the difference is due to the fact that the arterial pressure level is not high enough in some species to activate the baroceptor reflexes. Both baroceptor and chemoceptor activity in the sinus nerve have since been shown to be present after birth in a variety of mammals (kitten, rabbit, piglet, lamb and monkey).[20]

In 1954 Reynolds[21] expressed the prevailing opinion of that time as follows: "The view is now held that near term vagal tone develops in the fetus, and this is marked by a slow resting heart rate. Critical evaluation of the situation in new experiments in fetal lambs suggests, however, that there is no appreciable vagal tone in the fetus at rest before birth. However, the slightest degree of fetal circulatory distress induces demonstrable vagal tone. Similarly, there is no evidence of carotid sinus or sympathetic tone in the fetus, although activity over all these reflex pathways may be initiated by adequate stimulation."

The bulk of evidence thus far accumulated in the sheep suggests that the vasomotor reflexes are present in the fetus and become more sensitive during the latter part of pregnancy and after birth.[13-18,20-22] Recent studies indicate that contrary to earlier views the vasoconstrictor reflexes are present and functional at birth in the rabbit also.[23-25]

It is unlikely that the arterial pressure pattern observed beyond the neonatal period reflects a changing sensitivity of the vasomotor reflexes. The relationship of age to the sensitivity of these reflexes has been studied in older subjects but with conflicting results.[26,27]

Studies of the cardiac output in relation to age have been limited mainly to the fetus. Barcroft[16] found that the cardiac output in the sheep fetus increases with age. Studies in the human fetus, however, indicate that although the cardiac output increases progressively with weight, it remains constant when calculated on a unit weight basis.[28]

We postulate that beyond the neonatal period an increase in the cardiac output may be the major factor responsible for the increase in arterial pressure with growth. Since we were unable to find any recorded studies on this subject, the problem was approached indirectly by reviewing the available evidence relating to factors which are known to affect the cardiac output, i.e., stroke volume, heart rate, blood volume, blood viscosity and arterial elasticity.

The stroke volume increases and the heart rate decreases with age throughout all of childhood. Nylin[29] demonstrated in a longitudinal study that the stroke volume in humans increases with growth and with age. The heart rate, on the other hand, decreases with age. Others[30] found no sex differential in heart rate until about ten years of age at which time it decreases more rapidly in males than in females until about 15 years of age.

The total blood volume is known to increase as the body mass increases. The cellular elements are affected slightly more than the plasma so that the blood becomes more viscous with growth.[31,32] Coincident with the pubertal growth spurt, both blood volume and blood viscosity show a sharp rise, reaching a maximum in females at 13 years and in males at 17 years. It is of considerable interest that these ages are remarkably close to those for the maximum systolic arterial pressure.

When calculated on a unit basis, the increase in blood volume with growth is not so clear-cut as might be desired. Some studies indicate that unit blood volumes increase with an increase in weight;[33] others demonstrate an increase only when related to surface area;[32] and still others show an increase whether calculated on a weight or a surface area basis.[34] With sexual maturation both the blood viscosity and the blood volume tend to level off.[34-36] This suggests that the sex hormones may in some way be involved in the divergence of systolic arterial pressure in the two sexes at puberty. Evidence favoring this view has been presented by Lichton[4] and by Sturkie and Ringer[6] who demonstrated in chickens that the difference in arterial pressure between the two sexes is related to the output and/or utilization of pituitary gonadotropin.

It would seem reasonable to assume that the arterial tree becomes more rigid with age. Yet, little evidence could be found in the literature supporting this view. In fact, the two principal studies are contradictory in that Hallock and Benson[37] found in adults that the aorta becomes more rigid with age, but Remington and associates[38] found no correlation between absolute distensibility of the aorta and age.

From the somewhat confusing evidence at hand, it would appear that both cardiac output and peripheral vascular resistance account for the wide variation of arterial pressure observed in the newly born infant. Beyond this age period increases in cardiac output may well play the major role. Further research in this area is obviously needed. It is entirely possible that solution of the problems of blood pressure in childhood may be the key to the solution of hypertension in later life.

SUMMARY

Arterial pressure throughout the childhood years is characterized by a wide range of values in the early neonatal period followed by an almost uniform increase to the age of puberty. At puberty the systolic pressure reaches a maximum in females at about 12 years and in males at about 17 years of age.

The physiologic basis for these observations is obscure. It is postulated that the scatter of values peculiar to the early postnatal period is a reflection of changes in both peripheral vascular resistance and cardiac output; beyond this period and particularly at puberty an increase in the cardiac output may play the major role.

Data relating to these physiologic events remain inadequate, and the need for further research in this area is stressed.

REFERENCES

1. Tanner, J. M.: *Growth at Adolescence,* Springfield, Thomas, 1955.
2. Shock, N. W.: Basal blood pressure and pulse rate in adolescents, *Am. J. Dis. Child., 68*:16, 1944.
3. Clark, G. A.: Some foetal blood pressure reactions, *J. Physiol., 74*: 391, 1932.
4. Lichton, I. J.: Lack of normal blood pressure rise in growing chicken deprived of choline in early life, *Proc. Soc. Exp. Biol. and Med., 99*:634, 1958.
5. Sturkie, P. D., Weiss, H. S. and Ringer, R. K.: Effects of age on blood pressure in the chicken, *Am. J. Physiol., 174*:405, 1953.
6. Sturkie, P. D. and Ringer, R. K.: Effects of suppression of pituitary gonadotropins on blood pressure in the fowl, *Am. J. Physiol., 180*:53, 1955.
7. Weiss, H. S. and Sheahan, M.: Influence of maturity and sex on the blood pressure of the turkey, *Am. J. Vet. Res., 19*:209, 1958.
8. Cross, K. W., Dawes, G. S., and Mott, J. C.: Anoxia, oxygen consumption and cardiac output in newborn lambs and adult sheep. *J. Physiol., 146*:316, 1959.
9. Bauer, D. J.: Vagal reflexes appearing in asphyxia in rabbits at differenent ages, *J. Physiol., 95*:187, 1939.
10. Ringer, R. K., Weiss, H. S. and Sturkie, P. D.: Effect of sex and age on blood pressure in the duck and pigeon, *Am. J. Physiol., 183*:141, 1955.
11. Enhörnings, G. and Westin, B.: Experimental studies of the human fetus in prolonged asphyxia, Acta *Physiol. Scandinav., 31*:359, 1954.
12. Burlingame, P., Long, J. A., and Ogden, E.: The blood pressure of the fetal rat and its response to renin and augiotonin, *Am. J. Physiol., 137*:473, 1942.
13. Born, G. V. R., Dawes, G. S., and Mott, J. C.: Oxygen lack and autonomic nervous control of the foetal circulation in the lamb, *J. Physiol., 134*:149, 1956.
14. Barcroft, J. and Barron, D. H.: Blood pressure and pulse rate in foetal sheep, *J. Experim. Biol., 22*:63, 1945.
15. Born, G. V. R., Dawes, G. S., and Mott, J. C.: The viability of premature lambs, *J. Physiol., 130*:191, 1955.
16. Barcroft, J.: *Researches on Pre-Natal Life,* Springfield, Thomas, 1947.

17. Clark, G. A.: The development of blood pressure reflexes, *J. Physiol.*, *83*:229, 1934.

18. Bauer, D. J.: The slowing of heart rate produced by clamping the umbilical cord in the foetal sheep, *J. Physiol.*, *90*:25p,1937.

19. Bauer, D. J.: The effect of asphyxia upon the heart rate of rabbits at different ages, *J. Physiol.*, *93*:90, 1938.

20. Cross, K. W., and Malcolm, J. L.: Evidence of carotid body and sinus activity in new-born and foetal animals, *J. Physiol.*, *118*:10p,1952.

21. Reynolds, S. R. M.: Hemodynamic characteristics of the fetal circulation, *Am. J. Obst. & Gynec.*, *68*:69, 1954.

22. Dawes, G. S., Mott, J. C., and Rennick, B. R.: Some effects of adrenaline, noradrenaline and acetylcholine on the foetal circulation in the lamb, *J. Physiol.*, *134*:139, 1956.

23. Dawes, G. S., Handler, J. J., and Mott, J. C.: Some cardiovascular responses in foetal, new-born and adult rabbits, *J. Physiol.*, *139*:123, 1957.

24. Dawes, G. S.: Some respiratory and cardiovascular problems after birth, *Arch. Dis. Child.*, *34*:281, 1959.

25. Downing, S. E.: Baroreceptor reflexes in new-born rabbits, *J. Physiol.*, *150*:201, 1960.

26. Von Lottenbach, K., and Scharf, R.: Die pressorezeplorenfunktion und ihre beziehung zu alter und hochdruck, *Schweiz, Med. Woch.*, *87*:858, 1957.

27. Pickering, G. W., Kissin, M., and Rothschild, P.: The relationship of the carotid sinus mechanism to persistent high blood pressure in man, Clin. Sci. *Incorporating Heart, 2*:193, 1936.

28. Assali, N. S., Rauramo, L., and Peltonen, T.: Measurement of uterine blood flow and uterine metabolism. VIII. Uterine and fetal blood flow and oxygen consumption in early human pregnancy, *Am. J. Obst. & Gynec.*, *79*:86, 1960.

29. Nylin, G.: The physiology of the circulation during puberty, *Acta Med. Scandinav.*, Supp. 69, 1935.

30. Iliff, A., and Lee, V. A.: Pulse rate, respiratory rate, and body temperature of children between two months and eighteen years of age, *Child Development, 23*:238, 1952.

31. Gibson, J. G., Keeley, J. L., and Pijoan, M.: The blood volume of normal dogs, *Am. J. Physiol.*, *121*:800, 1938.

32. Russell, S. J. M.: Blood volume studies in healthy children, *Arch. Dis. Child.*, *24*:88, 1949.

33. Morse, M., Cassels, D. E., and Schultz, F. W.: Blood volumes of normal children, *Am. J. Physiol., 151*:448, 1947.
34. Brines, J. K., Gibson, J. G., and Kunkel, P.: The blood volume in normal infants and children, *J. Pediat., 18*:447, 1941.
35. Sjostrand, T.: Volume and distribution of blood and their significance in regulating circulation, *Physiol. Rev., 33*:202, 1953.
36. Mugrage, E. R., and Andresen, M. I.: Red blood cell values in adolescence, *Am. J. Dis. Child., 56*:997, 1938.
37. Hallock, P., and Benson, I. C.: Studies on the isolated properties of human isolated aorta, *J. Clin. Invest., 16*:595, 1937.
38. Remington, J. W., Noback, C. R., Hamilton, W. F., and Gold, J. J.: Volume elasticity characteristics of the human aorta and prediction of the stroke volume from the pressure pulse, *Am. J. Physiol. 153*:298, 1948.

INDEX